ABOUT THIS BOOK

This book contains four tailored workouts program for seniors. Each program is easy to follow since it has COLORED PICTURES FOR EACH EXERECISE, clear explanations of How to Perform Poses, suggestions To Avoid Common Mistakes and General Tips about each exercise.

You will find useful info about Pilates and its benefits, some nutrition advice and support for mental health. All the chapters in this book have been written to help you achieve optimum health and wellbeing.

You can practice one program at the time and when you feel comfortable with the exercises, move to the next one. The key to success with these Wall Pilates Program is to be patient, practice at your own pace and stay consistent, till you are ready to complete a 28-days program.

What is 28-days program? It will be explained in the next chapters.

If you have any question, you can contact me at:
ritadavis.pilates@gmail.com

DISCLAIMER

This information is for your personal use ONLY. You cannot distribute, copy, reproduce, or otherwise sell this product or information in any form whatsoever, including but not limited to: electronic, or mechanical, including photocopying, recording, or by any informational storage or retrieval system without expressed written, dated and signed permission from the author. All copyrights are reserved.

The information, including but not limited to, text, graphics, images and other material contained in this guide are for informational purposes only. No material from this guide is intended to be a substitute for professional medical advice, diagnosis or treatment.

Always seek the advice of your physician or other qualified health care provider with any questions you may have regarding a medical condition or treatment and before undertaking a new health care regimen, and never disregard professional medical advice or delay in seeking it because of something you have read in this guide.

**"Take care of your body.
It's the only place where you have to live!"**

Jim Rohn

TABLE OF CONTENTS

INTRODUCTION

Wall Pilates is a unique form of exercise that originated in Germany during the late 19th century. It was developed by Joseph H. Pilates, who believed that the physical, mental and spiritual elements of the body should all be connected and in harmony with one another.

Joseph Pilates was a pioneer of his time and wanted to create an exercise that focused on improving strength, posture and flexibility. He developed Wall Pilates as a combination of western and eastern exercise disciplines that focused on targeting the body's deep muscles, connecting them to each other and strengthening them as one unit.

Unlike the typical mat-based Pilates class, wall Pilates uses wall bars to give an even more precise approach to strengthening and sculpting the body. It focuses on pushing and pulling exercises and movement drills which helps create balance, power, agility and stamina. This approach helps to engage the body's core muscles, enhance muscular coordination and create fluid, controlled movements.

By targeting the body's smaller muscles with wall Pilates, it also helps improve posture, boost energy levels and helps reduce aches and pains. It also creates long lasting body changes and improved quality of movement that you can carry with you through everyday activities and workouts.

Joseph Pilates developed wall Pilates more than 100 years ago, but the unique approach and benefits it offers to those who practice it have made it increasingly popular around the world.

The goal of this book is not just to help you learn and understand more about wall Pilates, but to also help you become healthier by getting you to move. Your wellbeing is very important to us, and we want to make sure that you have everything you need to maintain your independence through the golden years. With the information we share with you in this book, you're going to fall back in love with your body, mind and health. You're going to live a healthier and more fulfilling life. And this is what it's all about. We only live once, and we have to make it count.

AUTHOR BIO

Rita Davis is a personal trainer with over 20 years of experience who specializes in senior workouts and has a passion for Nutrition, Yoga, Pilates, and Mindfulness. Rita has dedicated her career to helping seniors stay healthy and active through safe and effective exercise programs and personalized nutrition plans.

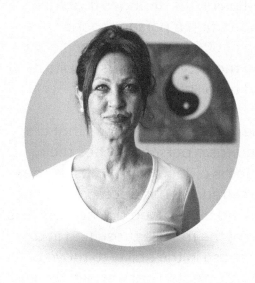

In addition to her work as a personal trainer, Rita is an experienced Pilates and Yoga instructor who incorporates exercises into her clients' workouts to improve their strength, flexibility, and posture.

Rita's passion for health and wellness extends beyond fitness. She provides her clients with valuable nutrition advice and guidance to support their fitness goals. In her free time, practices mindfulness, which she believes is essential for managing stress and promoting overall well-being.

CHANGES AS WE AGE

As the human body ages, many significant changes can occur. In particular, the changes that take place when a person reaches the age of 60 or above are significant and may impact a person's lifestyle and mobility.

One of the main changes that can occur as a person reaches their sixties is a decrease in muscle mass and strength. This decrease can be caused by reduced activity and less use of the muscles, resulting in a decrease in the ability to move or lift heavy objects. Furthermore, the joints become less flexible, which makes moving or bending more difficult. This may make performing everyday tasks more difficult.

The bones also start to become weaker, with bones becoming more brittle as a person ages. This can lead to a greater risk of fractures, particularly when the bones become weaker or when there is an underlying condition such as osteoporosis.

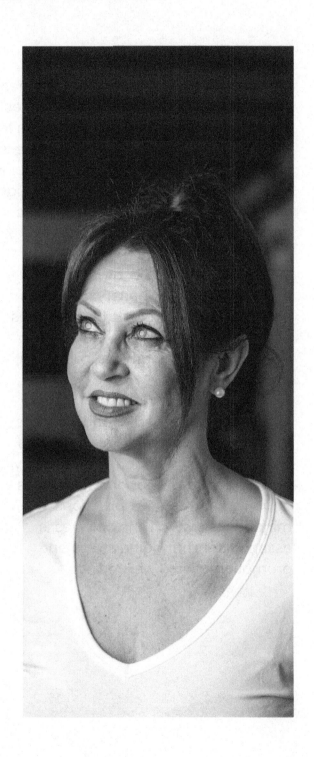

Another physical change that often occurs is the decrease in lung capacity, resulting in shortness of breath and an increase in coughing. This may be caused by an increase in conditions such as COPD and other age-related respiratory problems.

Skin elasticity is also greatly affected, as the production of collagen slows down as we age, resulting in skin that is more prone to wrinkles, age spots and other blemishes.

It is also common for vision and hearing to decline as people get older, which may make it more difficult to complete certain tasks or participate in activities.

Finally, the immune system starts to weaken, making people more vulnerable to illnesses, infections, and diseases. As a result, people aged 60 or above may need to take extra precautions and steps to protect themselves.

Overall, as a person ages, their body can undergo significant changes, with those aged 60 or above being particularly susceptible to physical and medical changes. It is important to remain active, to take necessary precautions and steps, and to monitor your health in order to help mitigate any negative effects that these changes can bring.

"Exercise not only keeps us fit, but gives us strength, stamina and spirit. Stay active, stay healthy and make your senior years your golden years!"

WHAT IS WALL PILATES?

Wall Pilates is an effective, low-impact form of exercise designed to help strengthen, stretch, and balance the body. It's ideal for those looking to add an extra dimension of physical activity to their routine. Wall Pilates involves using the wall for resistance in a wide variety of different poses and movements.

A typical Wall Pilates class may include a variety of poses that challenge the entire body, from simple stretches to intense exercises. Common movements can include: push-ups, hip thrusts, sit-ups, planks, stretches, balance poses, and more. In addition, exercises can be tailored to fit your personal needs and fitness goals.

Wall Pilates is suitable for all ages and can be adjusted to suit each person's ability level. For seniors over 60, Wall Pilates is an excellent form of exercise, as it's gentle and can be tailored to any age or ability. This low-impact form of exercise has numerous benefits such as improving posture, flexibility, and strength, and reducing stress and fatigue. Additionally, seniors may be more likely to continue the routine with Wall Pilates, as it requires little equipment and can be done at the convenience of their own home.

If you are looking for a safe, effective way to get your body moving, then wall Pilates might be the perfect choice for you. As we grow older, we start to understand the effects of our younger days on our health and wellbeing. Some choices may have been great, while others should have been avoided. Whatever choices we made early in the days can determine how mobile we are in our golden years. So, understanding the importance of our health and wellbeing, we wrote this book. The purpose of it is not to sell you anything special, it's to guide you through workout routines that will help you feel stronger, happier and more independent. We are here every step of the way.

Over the next few pages, you'll learn more about wall Pilates and how to make the most of your exercise.

HOW EFFECTIVE IS WALL PILATES?

Wall Pilates is a growing exercise trend that utilizes an exercise wall, or sling wall, as part of the workout. The practice focuses on improving flexibility, coordination, strength, and balance with wall-assisted movement, rather than floor-based exercises. Proponents of this approach argue that it offers an accessible and gentle introduction to Pilates for those new to the discipline.

Origins of Wall Pilates can be traced back to Germany in the late 1920s, when Joseph Pilates created his famous exercises with the help of pulley systems suspended from walls and ceilings. Since then, this wall-assisted exercise has been studied extensively, with some researchers arguing that it can offer therapeutic benefits in various contexts, including the elderly and post-rehabilitative care.

In terms of therapeutic benefits, wall Pilates is said to have an impact on the improvement of strength, flexibility, and mobility, as well as providing relief from back pain. There have been a number of studies that have focused on the efficacy of wall Pilates in helping people of all ages, fitness levels, and abilities, as well as those who are undergoing physical rehabilitation.

Wall Pilates is also known to improve coordination and balance, due to the focus on dynamic movements and changing positions while using the wall to support and challenge. Additionally, by engaging multiple body parts simultaneously, the practice helps with joint flexibility, strength, and endurance, as well as helping to reduce tension in the shoulders and hips.

Given the popularity of Pilates in general, wall Pilates has the potential to be widely adopted as an alternative form of exercise, as well as offering rehabilitation benefits for a range of physical needs. Although there is a need for further research in order to determine the specific effects and applications of wall Pilates, it has already been established that the practice offers many benefits for people of all fitness levels.

WHY IS WALL PILATES GOOD FOR SENIORS?

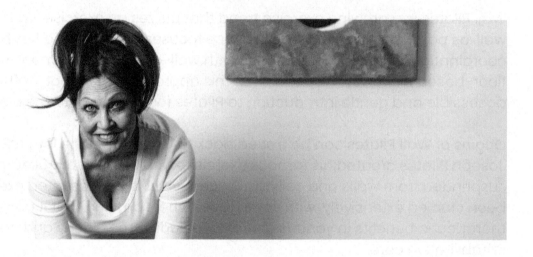

Wall Pilates is a fantastic form of exercise for seniors as it provides them with the ability to get their body moving, stay strong and healthy, and experience increased energy levels. This low-impact exercise can be adapted to each individual's ability and allows for modified postures and intensity of exercises. Wall Pilates is ideal for older adults because it focuses on balance, core strength, and proper body alignment, which can all be beneficial in terms of physical fitness and independence.

Wall Pilates encourages seniors to use all of the muscles in their body as opposed to isolated movements that may focus on certain muscles groups. The routine of wall Pilates is often different each day and can include challenging, yet rewarding, exercises that work multiple parts of the body. Furthermore, because it's an isometric exercise that requires minimal motion, seniors can practice wall Pilates safely, making it an ideal form of exercise for those with arthritis, mobility impairments, and other age-related issues.

Moreover, wall Pilates can help increase energy and overall strength for seniors. By focusing on muscular endurance, balance, and stability, wall Pilates increases core strength, making everyday activities like walking, climbing stairs, and getting in and out of a chair more efficient and easier. It also helps improve flexibility and range of motion, so seniors can enjoy an increased ability to perform their everyday activities.

In addition to its physical benefits, wall Pilates also has a calming effect. It increases seniors' awareness of their breathing, which helps lower stress levels, promote relaxation, and reduce anxiety. Moreover, the controlled movements required in wall Pilates can provide seniors with a feeling of control and mastery of their own body, increasing their sense of physical autonomy and psychological well-being.

Overall, wall Pilates can be an excellent form of exercise for seniors who want to remain healthy and independent. With its low impact exercises, controlled movements, and beneficial health benefits, wall Pilates can help seniors increase their energy and physical ability, improve their mental and emotional state, and boost their overall quality of life.

BENEFITS OF WALL PILATES

Wall Pilates is an exercise system that has become increasingly popular over the past decade. It's a unique form of Pilates that utilizes the support of a wall to provide stability and resistance to help improve overall strength and mobility. This form of exercise provides numerous physical and mental benefits, many of which may surprise you. In this chapter, we'll take a closer look at the 10 surprising health benefits of wall Pilates.

STRENGTHENS THE FULL BODY

Wall Pilates is an excellent full body workout. It engages and strengthens all major muscle groups, from your shoulders and arms to your core, legs, and feet. The wall provides a stable surface for you to press into, which engages the muscles in a way that other forms of exercise cannot. This can help you develop strength and definition in your body more quickly and efficiently than traditional workouts.

Plus, the exercises are easy to modify based on your current fitness level. So, whether you're a beginner or a more advanced exerciser, wall pilates can help you reach your goals.

Wall pilates can help strengthen your muscles and improve their tone, making them look toned and defined. And since these exercises are low-impact, they're less likely to cause any strain or injury on your joints.

IMPROVES POSTURE

One of the most notable health benefits of wall Pilates is improved posture. By regularly performing wall Pilates exercises, you can improve your posture and stand taller. That's because wall Pilates strengthens and tones muscles in the core, back, and abdomen that are used for good posture.

Wall Pilates also helps to promote flexibility in the spine, which further contributes to better posture. Regularly performing wall Pilates exercises can help to strengthen weak muscles and stretch tight ones. This can improve your posture over time and help you stand taller with confidence.

In addition, wall Pilates helps with posture by promoting good spinal alignment. This is especially true when you perform the wall Pilates leg exercises. These exercises involve pushing the lower back into the wall while engaging the abdominal muscles to maintain a neutral spine position. This allows you to keep your spine straight and maintain good posture while performing the exercises.

Overall, wall Pilates can be a great way to improve your posture and keep it looking its best. Regularly performing these exercises will not only help you to stand taller, but also help your muscles stay strong and healthy. So if you're looking for an easy way to improve your posture, give wall Pilates a try!

STRENGTHENS THE CORE

Pilates is known for its core strengthening benefits, and wall pilates is no exception. Wall pilates will help to strengthen the core muscles, such as the abdominal muscles, back muscles, and hip muscles.

Doing wall pilates regularly can help to build stronger core muscles, which can improve overall body stability and strength. It can also help to reduce the risk of injury during everyday activities. Working out on the wall will also help to stretch and tone the abdominal muscles, providing support for the lower back and improving posture.

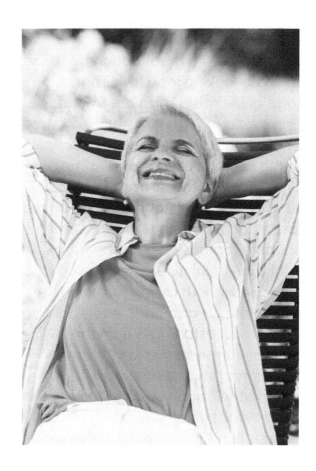

TONES THE ARMS AND LEGS

If you're looking to tone your arms and legs, Wall Pilates is an effective way to do it. The exercises in Wall Pilates are designed to target your major muscle groups and help you build strength. For example, one of the main moves is a pike press. To do this, you stand facing the wall, place both hands on the wall, and then slowly lift your body up and down. This move helps to target your arms, chest, and legs, helping you to tone and sculpt those areas. You can also do other moves like wall squats, which helps to target your legs and glutes. Through regular practice of Wall Pilates, you'll start to see toned muscles in no time!

LOW-IMPACT WORKOUT

Wall Pilates is a great option for those who are looking for a low-impact form of exercise. This type of Pilates can be done with minimal equipment, allowing you to practice it in the comfort of your own home. Unlike many other forms of exercise, Wall Pilates does not put stress on the joints and ligaments. This makes it suitable for those who suffer from joint pain or injury as they can still exercise without risking further injury. Wall Pilates is also perfect for those who are just starting out on their fitness journey as it allows them to build strength and tone up without putting their body through too much strain. Wall Pilates is a great way to get a full-body workout with minimal risk of injury.

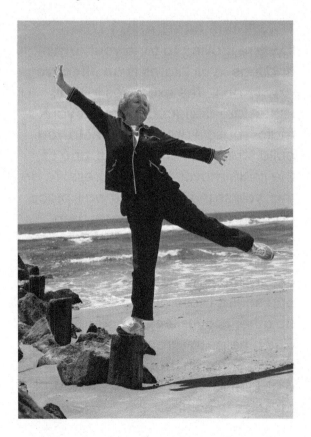

CAN HELP WITH WEIGHT LOSS

Wall Pilates is a great way to shed unwanted pounds. The moves are designed to engage and work your core muscles, which helps burn more calories. Wall Pilates also increases your heart rate while keeping your joints safe from harm. This means that you get a great workout without putting undue strain on your body. In addition, Wall Pilates can help build muscle tone and definition in the arms, legs, and core. This makes it easier to create the calorie deficit needed for weight loss. With the right routine and diet, Wall Pilates can help you reach your weight loss goals.

IMPROVES BALANCE AND COORDINATION

Pilates is well known for its ability to improve coordination and balance, and wall Pilates is no different. With wall Pilates, you can challenge your body to stabilize while using multiple muscles in a coordinated fashion. This helps to improve your balance and coordination, making everyday activities like walking, running, or sports much easier. You'll be able to move with more agility and accuracy, thanks to the improved balance and coordination that wall Pilates provides. Wall Pilates can also help improve your reflexes, which can come in handy for sports or even just performing everyday tasks like opening a door or carrying a grocery bag. If you're looking for a great way to improve your balance and coordination, wall Pilates is definitely worth a try!

GREAT STRESS RELIEVER

Exercising can help reduce stress levels, and Wall Pilates is no exception. Because Wall Pilates is low-impact and uses the wall as support, you don't need to worry about strain or injury during your workout. This allows you to relax and focus on the movement and breathing patterns, which can help you let go of any tension and stress. Additionally, Wall Pilates can help improve your posture, which in turn can reduce stress in your body. The combination of deep breathing and controlled movement can also help release endorphins, which can help improve your mood and reduce stress. So if you're looking for a way to de-stress, Wall Pilates is a great option!

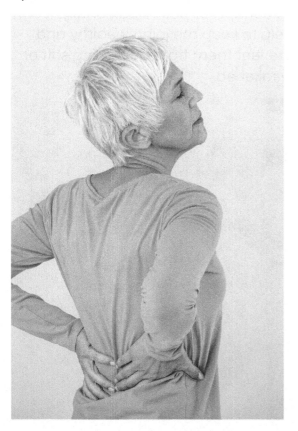

CAN HELP IMPROVE SLEEP

Studies show that regular exercise, such as Wall Pilates, can improve sleep quality. When we exercise, our body temperature increases and when it drops, it signals our body to become sleepy. Regular exercise can also reduce stress and fatigue, both of which are major causes of insomnia. Additionally, Wall Pilates helps to relax the mind and body, which can be beneficial for falling asleep and staying asleep. Finally, Wall Pilates is a gentle form of exercise that is not overly strenuous, so it won't interfere with your sleep if done before bedtime. All in all, Wall Pilates can be a great way to help improve your overall sleep quality.

CAN HELP RELIEVE BACK PAIN

Back pain is an all-too-common problem that affects people of all ages and walks of life. Thankfully, Wall Pilates offers a low-impact solution that can help relieve back pain. By strengthening your core muscles, improving your posture, and allowing you to move in a more controlled and mindful way, Wall Pilates can be an effective tool in managing and even eliminating back pain.

Wall Pilates allows you to move slowly and with precision while focusing on your breath, which can be incredibly calming for your mind and body. When you're focusing on your breath and your body alignment, you'll be able to identify the areas of tension in your back and work to release it.

Wall Pilates also strengthens your core muscles which supports your spine and helps keep your posture aligned. This increases stability and flexibility in the spine and reduces pressure on the lower back. A strong core also helps improve balance, making everyday activities easier and reducing strain on the lower back.

Wall Pilates can also help to stretch the muscles in your back and realign your vertebrae. Stretching helps increase blood flow to the muscles, which is essential for recovery.

Overall, Wall Pilates can be an effective tool in helping to reduce or even eliminate back pain. By strengthening your core, improving posture, increasing flexibility, and allowing you to move with precision and focus, Wall Pilates can help restore balance to your mind and body and bring relief from back pain.

REDUCES TIGHTNESS AND SORENESS IN MUSCLES

Wall Pilates is great for reducing tension and soreness in the muscles. This is because it works all of the major muscle groups and helps to improve circulation and range of motion. As you do the exercises, you will be able to stretch the muscles and release any built-up tension and soreness that may have accumulated throughout the day. This can help reduce chronic pain as well as make it easier to move around and do activities without feeling stiff or uncomfortable. Wall Pilates is a great way to relax the body and improve overall flexibility.

REDUCES SORENESS IN JOINTS AND LIGAMENTS

One of the best things about wall pilates is that it can reduce tightness and soreness in both your joints and ligaments. Pilates' combination of stretching and strengthening exercises works to realign your body, reducing the strain and pressure on your joints and ligaments. This means that wall pilates can help to keep you feeling limber and mobile. By doing regular wall pilates exercises, you can maintain healthy flexibility in your joints, allowing you to move freely and enjoy activities with less discomfort or pain. Additionally, it can help to keep the joints healthy and prevent them from becoming stiff or weakened.

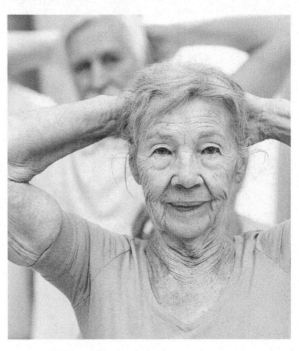

INCREASES FLEXIBILITY

Flexibility is an important part of physical health, and wall pilates can help with this. Wall pilates helps to lengthen the muscles, increase range of motion, and improve joint mobility. Regular practice of wall pilates can help you become more flexible and better able to perform everyday activities. Wall pilates also encourages proper form and technique, which can help reduce the risk of injury. Stretching is also important in wall pilates to help further increase flexibility. With consistent practice, you will begin to feel the benefits of increased flexibility in your body and movements.

IMPROVES CONFIDENCE AND SELF-ESTEEM

Wall Pilates is a great way to help increase your confidence and self-esteem. The increased strength, flexibility and balance that comes with wall pilates helps boost your confidence. Wall Pilates also helps improve your body awareness and posture, which can have a huge impact on how you feel about yourself. When you see your body getting stronger and more toned, it can be incredibly empowering and help boost your self-esteem. The sense of accomplishment that comes with mastering the wall pilates moves can also help build your confidence and self-esteem.

BUILDS RESILIENCE

Resilience is defined as the ability to bounce back from stress and adapt to difficult situations. Wall pilates can help to build resilience in the body and mind by improving physical endurance, strength, and flexibility. Pilates helps you become stronger, both physically and mentally, allowing you to handle difficult situations better. With regular wall pilates practice, you will be able to increase your resistance to fatigue and build up your ability to tolerate more strenuous activity. Wall pilates also helps reduce mental stress and improve concentration, enabling you to focus better on challenging tasks. As a result, wall pilates can help you build up your resilience so that you are better able to handle life's stresses and challenges.

IMPROVES MOOD

Wall Pilates can be a great way to improve your overall mood. Studies have shown that regular physical activity can increase endorphins and serotonin in the brain, leading to improved mood and lower levels of depression and anxiety. Wall Pilates is an excellent form of low-impact exercise that can help you get the same benefits without overexerting yourself. As you start to practice wall pilates regularly, you may find yourself feeling happier and more relaxed as your body gets stronger and more flexible. Not only can Wall Pilates improve your mood, but it can also give you a sense of accomplishment and self-confidence as you progress and perfect your technique.

DEVELOPS MINDFULNESS

Mindfulness is an important factor in achieving overall wellness. Wall pilates helps to cultivate mindfulness by having the participant focus on each movement and exercise, allowing them to become aware of their body and how it moves. Wall Pilates encourages the participant to keep their breathing steady and controlled during each exercise and movement, which helps to center the mind and relax the body. It also helps to develop awareness of body alignment and posture, which helps to improve coordination and balance. By practicing mindfulness during wall pilates, participants can gain a deeper understanding of their body and how it works, as well as how to move efficiently and with proper form. As a result, this practice can help to reduce mental stress and anxiety, as well as physical stress from everyday activities.

IMPROVES INDEPENDENCE

Wall Pilates is an excellent form of exercise for seniors. The low-impact nature of the exercise allows seniors to practice without putting strain on their joints or muscles. Wall Pilates helps strengthen the core muscles and improve balance, which can help seniors move with greater confidence and ease. Additionally, Wall Pilates can also improve mobility, allowing seniors to enjoy activities they may have given up due to limited physical abilities. With regular practice, seniors can gain increased independence as they are able to move more confidently and with less assistance. Wall Pilates is also a great way for seniors to increase their flexibility and reduce stiffness in their bodies. Lastly, wall pilates can help improve mood and reduce stress, which can contribute to a better overall quality of life for seniors.

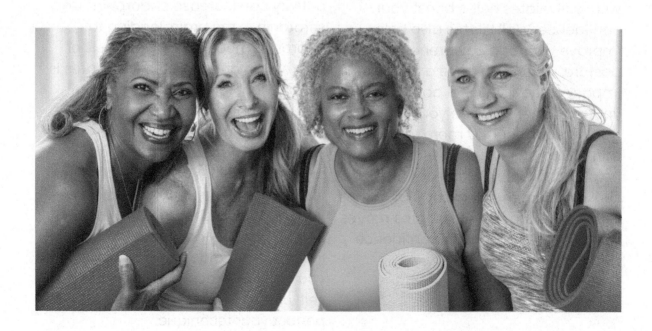

CAN AID IN PHYSICAL REHABILITATION

Wall pilates is a great form of exercise for people who are recovering from an injury or dealing with chronic pain. The low-impact nature of wall pilates makes it a safe and effective form of exercise for those looking to get back on their feet after an injury or surgery.

Wall pilates can help increase flexibility and range of motion, while also helping to reduce tightness and soreness in muscles, joints and ligaments. By strengthening the muscles and stabilizing the joints, wall pilates can help improve movement patterns and reduce the risk of re-injury.

Wall pilates can also help with postural alignment and balance, both of which are important for physical rehabilitation. By targeting specific muscles groups, wall pilates helps improve overall stability and coordination, allowing individuals to move more confidently with less risk of injury.

Overall, wall pilates is a great way for people to get back on their feet after an injury or surgery. Whether you're looking to build strength, improve flexibility or rehabilitate from an injury, wall pilates is a great option that can help you reach your goals.

REDUCES DEPRESSION AND ANXIETY

Depression and anxiety can take a toll on your mental health, but practicing wall pilates may help. Wall pilates is an excellent way to relax your body and mind, which in turn can help reduce stress levels and symptoms of depression and anxiety. It allows you to focus on the present moment instead of worrying about the future or ruminating about the past. The deep breathing and stretching that come with wall pilates can help clear the mind and reduce tension in the body. By releasing stress, endorphins are released, helping to elevate your mood. Wall pilates also helps to reduce negative self-talk, providing a positive reinforcement to your thoughts and actions.

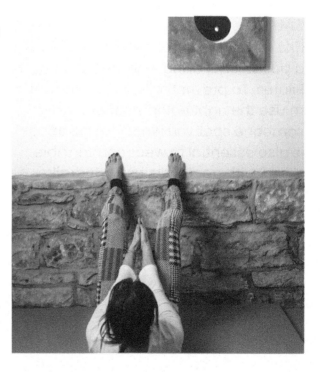

PRECAUTIONS

Wall Pilates can be a great exercise for seniors to help maintain strength, flexibility, and balance. However, it's important to be aware of the potential dangers that come with the practice. As with any form of physical activity, there are certain risks involved, especially when it comes to senior citizens. In this chapter, we'll explore certain potential dangers of Wall Pilates and discuss how to safely practice the exercise. From ensuring proper form to understanding the limitations of your body, we'll cover all the essential tips to help you stay safe and healthy.

FALLS

Like with any type of exercise, falling is a possibility. Falling while performing Pilates. To prevent falls, it is important to use the right equipment and have someone spot you when necessary. It is also essential to wear comfortable shoes with good grip, use handrails, and practice the moves in a well-lit area. Additionally, if you feel dizzy or unsteady during your session, it is best to stop and rest before continuing.

BROKEN BONES

Seniors who are unfamiliar with the moves or who have weakened bones and muscles should take extra care when performing wall Pilates. A sudden movement or incorrect form can result in an uncontrolled movement that can cause a fall or injury. Not that broken bones are common, but it is a possibility.

Before beginning wall Pilates, be aware of your own limits and strengths. You should always consult a physician before beginning any exercise program. If possible, work with an experienced trainer who can ensure you are performing the exercises correctly and within your abilities.

When performing wall Pilates, take care to move slowly and deliberately, as sudden or jerky movements can put extra pressure and weight on your bones and joints which can cause a broken bone. Ensure you exercise proper form too. This means keeping your spine aligned and maintaining good posture during each exercise. Additionally, make sure to choose appropriate exercises that match your strength and ability level.

MUSCLE STRAINS

One of the most common risks is muscle strains. These happen when the muscles are overworked or stretched beyond their normal range of motion. This can be especially dangerous for seniors because they may not have the same amount of flexibility as younger people.

To help prevent muscle strains, you should always perform Wall Pilates exercises slowly and carefully. Take frequent breaks to allow the muscles to rest and recover. We both know how exciting it is to start a new endeavor, especially if it all about bettering yourself. But, by giving yourself time and rest, you are ensuring the sustainability of the program.

One thing that many people often overlook is listening to their body cues. If they are tired, they will still exercise or try to 'power through' their day. However, doing these kinds of actions on regular basis and forgetting that your body NEEDS care, time and rest is only going to backfire over long term. So, take care of yourself. Listen to your body and make sure you work in partnership with it, and not against it.

JOINT INJURIES

Performing wall Pilates can carry a slight risk of joint injuries, which can occur from overstretching. When stretching during wall Pilates, it's important to know your body's limitations and not to push yourself beyond what you can safely handle. It is especially important to make sure that you keep your knees, hips, shoulders, elbows, wrists and ankles in proper alignment during each exercise to prevent any joint pain or injury. Additionally, be mindful of the movements you are making and be aware of any pain or discomfort you may be feeling in your joints. If you experience pain while performing wall Pilates, stop immediately and contact a medical professional.

HEAD INJURIES

Head injuries can be particularly dangerous for seniors. The sudden and intense movements can cause the head to hit against the wall, resulting in a serious injury. To prevent this from happening, make sure that there is plenty of space for your exercise poses and to protect yourself, add some cushions around your training space. This can help to protect you and your head.

HEART ATTACKS

As we age, our heart is a little more susceptible to heart problems and heart disease. So, when performing an y type of exercise, make sure not to push yourself too much.

Cardiovascular exercise, such as wall Pilates, can be beneficial for heart health in many ways, however, it is important to be mindful of any underlying heart issues that you may have. If you've had or have a heart condition, be sure to speak to a physician prior to performing wall Pilates to ensure it is safe for you.

If you are ready to get started but you care cautious about your cardiovascular health, make sure to take regular breaks, drink plenty of fluids and pay attention to your body's signals. If you experience any pain, tightness in the chest or difficulty breathing, stop and seek medical attention immediately as these can be signs of a heart attack. Additionally, it is important to not over-exert yourself when performing wall Pilates and to slowly build up endurance to avoid pushing the body beyond its limits.

HEAT EXHAUSTION

Wall Pilates can be a great form of exercise for seniors, but it is important to be aware of the dangers of heat exhaustion. This can happen when you overexert yourself in an environment that is too hot, or if you are wearing heavy clothing. Symptoms of heat exhaustion include excessive sweating, dizziness, confusion, and fatigue. If these symptoms occur, it is important to take a break and move to a cooler area. It is also important to drink plenty of fluids and replace electrolytes. If symptoms persist, it is important to seek medical attention immediately.

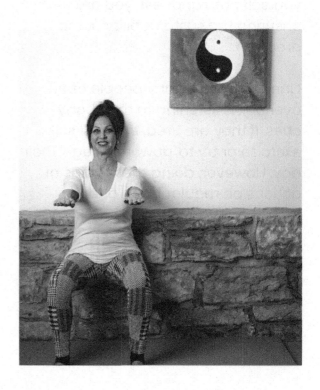

DEHYDRATION

When engaging in any exercise, it's important to stay hydrated and keep an eye out for signs of dehydration. In general, you should always keep a bottle of water nearby when performing exercise and take frequent breaks for drinking and resting. Common signs of dehydration include dry mouth, dark urine, fatigue, dizziness, confusion, headaches, and irritability. If any of these symptoms are present, you should immediately stop exercising and drink plenty of fluids to replenish electrolytes and prevent further health complications.

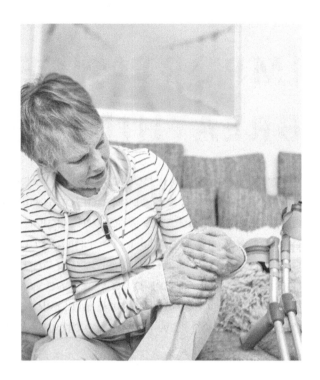

CRAMPS

Cramps can occur when performing wall Pilates, especially in seniors. When muscles are overworked, they become tight and may cramp up, leading to pain and discomfort. This is due to the lack of oxygen getting to the muscles, which prevents them from releasing lactic acid that builds up during exercise. To prevent cramps, take frequent breaks throughout your workout, use a foam roller to relax the muscles, and drink plenty of fluids before and after your session. Stretching both before and after exercising can also help loosen tight muscles and reduce the likelihood of experiencing cramps.

RHABDOMYOLYSIS

Rhabdomyolysis is a rare, but serious condition that can occur when performing exercise. It occurs when muscle tissue breaks down and the proteins and electrolytes released into the bloodstream can cause kidney damage. Symptoms of rhabdomyolysis include extreme fatigue, muscle pain, weakness, dark colored urine, fever, confusion, rapid heart rate, and nausea. If these symptoms are experienced, it is important to seek medical attention immediately. To reduce the risk of rhabdomyolysis, it is important to properly warm up and cool down before and after wall Pilates exercises, as well as to drink plenty of fluids before, during, and after the workout.

IMPORTANCE OF BREATHING

As we get older, our bodies naturally become less flexible and more prone to injury. Therefore, it is essential for seniors to be mindful of the way they move and take precautions when engaging in physical activity, especially during wall pilates. Proper breathing technique can help ensure that seniors remain safe and comfortable while exercising and can even enhance the effectiveness of their workouts. In this blog post, we will discuss the importance of proper breathing for seniors during wall pilates and exercise in general. We will also provide tips on how to ensure proper breathing during physical activity.

WHAT IS PROPER BREATHING?

Proper breathing is a type of conscious, mindful breathing that has numerous physical and mental health benefits. It helps regulate the body's vital functions such as heart rate, digestion, and oxygenation of tissues and organs. Proper breathing also helps reduce stress and anxiety, as well as improve sleep quality.

When it comes to exercise, proper breathing is essential for maximizing the benefits of the activity. When performing Wall Pilates and other forms of exercise, proper breathing techniques help maximize oxygen intake while strengthening and stretching the body. Proper breathing techniques also help increase focus, coordination, and balance during the activity.

When breathing properly during Wall Pilates and other exercises, it is important to inhale deeply through the nose and exhale slowly through the mouth. This type of mindful breathing helps bring oxygen to the muscles and organs in order to promote physical and mental relaxation. It also helps ensure that the body does not become overly stressed or fatigued during exercise.

THE DANGERS OF POOR BREATHING TECHNIQUES

It is important for seniors to practice proper breathing techniques when doing any type of exercise, especially wall pilates. Poor breathing can lead to a number of dangers for seniors. For example, it can cause shallow breathing which leads to low oxygen levels in the body. This can then cause fatigue and an increased heart rate, both of which can be dangerous for seniors. Additionally, improper breathing can cause hyperventilation and dizziness, which can also lead to accidents. Lastly, poor breathing can lead to muscle strain and fatigue, both of which can be painful and debilitating.

For these reasons, it is important for seniors to practice proper breathing techniques when engaging in any type of exercise. Not only will proper breathing help to avoid the aforementioned dangers, it will also help seniors achieve maximum benefit from their workouts. Proper breathing helps to increase oxygen levels in the body, improve endurance and increase circulation. All of these things can be beneficial for seniors as they engage in exercise.

THE BENEFITS OF PROPER BREATHING

When seniors practice proper breathing during Wall Pilates and other exercises, they can experience a number of health benefits. Proper breathing helps to maintain a healthy heart rate, reduce stress and anxiety, improve energy levels, and even help boost your mood.

Proper breathing also helps seniors maintain optimal blood pressure and oxygen levels. When you breathe properly during exercise, you are able to access more oxygen, which can help your body work more efficiently. This can help reduce fatigue and improve your performance during Wall Pilates and other exercises.

Breathing correctly can also help increase the range of motion in seniors' joints, which can lead to better balance and coordination. Proper breathing techniques can also help alleviate pain caused by conditions such as arthritis, as well as back pain due to poor posture or aging.

Finally, proper breathing techniques can help seniors to relax their mind and body and improve mental clarity. Taking slow deep breaths can have a calming effect on the nervous system, helping to promote better sleep and reduce stress.

TIPS FOR PROPER BREATHING WHILE DOING PILATES

CONCENTRATE ON YOUR BREATHING

Before you start a Pilates exercise, make sure to take some time to focus on your breathing. Take a few moments to inhale and exhale deeply, allowing your body to relax and concentrate on your breath.

PRACTICE RHYTHMIC BREATHING

As you do Pilates exercises, focus on making your inhalations and exhalations in a smooth, consistent rhythm. This will help you maintain control of your movements as well as your breathing.

COORDINATE WITH MOVEMENTS

When you're doing a Pilates exercise, coordinate your movements with your breath. For example, when doing the bridge exercise, inhale before lifting your hips off the floor and then exhale as you lift them.

KEEP YOUR CORE ENGAGED

Throughout your Pilates exercises, keep your core muscles engaged by drawing in your abdominal muscles and slightly lifting up through your ribcage while keeping your shoulders down. This will help you maintain proper breathing form and prevent you from hunching over or slouching.

BE MINDFUL

When you're doing Pilates, it's important to be aware of your breath. Don't rush through exercises or forget to breathe altogether. Listen to your body and don't forget to take breaks if you need them.

By following these tips, you can make sure that you're properly breathing while doing Pilates exercises. Proper breathing is an essential part of staying safe and maximizing the benefits of Pilates for seniors. With practice and dedication, you can soon be reaping the rewards of proper breathing and enjoying all the benefits Pilates has to offer.

YOUR COMMITMENT

Committing to yourself is an essential part of any successful health and wellness journey. This commitment involves both dedication and motivation to stay on track and continue making progress towards achieving your desired goals.

With tailored exercises and personalized instruction, our 28-day Wall Pilates program helps you learn proper technique to optimize the effectiveness of your movements.

Performing wall Pilates can make a world of difference in staying committed to your health and wellness. Through simple routines, you'll have access to step-by-step instructions and detailed pictures of each exercise. Get your partner involved to create a sense of competition! Even in golden years, we enjoy being stronger than our other half.

In addition to providing guidance and support, Wall Pilates provides accountability, making sure you are consistently doing your best to move forward and reach your goals. This can mean a lot when you're struggling to stay motivated and stay on track. When you feel like giving up, having a consistent plan of action and the accountability to complete it can help keep you going.

Finally, committing to yourself and Wall Pilates allows you to be proud of your progress and your accomplishments. Celebrating your successes along the way is important in developing healthy habits and staying motivated. Wall Pilates also offers performance tracking which helps you recognize when you're making progress and gaining strength, as well as when you need to tweak something in order to keep progressing.

When you make a commitment to yourself and to Wall Pilates, you're taking charge of your health and well-being and making sure you have the best tools available to reach your goals.

WHAT DO YOU NEED TO GET STARTED

Getting started couldn't be easier. Wall Pilates doesn't require any fancy equipment or a lot of space. That's what makes it so perfect. If you're a senior looking for an exercise program that can improve your strength and mobility, then Pilates is a great choice! This low-impact exercise system has become popular among people of all ages. Senior citizens who have started doing Pilates can expect improved core strength, improved balance, better posture, increased flexibility and improved coordination.

The great thing about Pilates is that it doesn't require any expensive equipment or fancy classes, which makes it accessible to anyone of all abilities. With our 28-day wall Pilates program, you're going to receive everything you need from instructional images to step-by step instructions. So, we take away the guess work. All you need is simple equipment to make you feel more comfortable and safe during movements. To get started, you will need the following:

- A Mat: Invest in a good quality mat. You'll be using it often and for long periods of time, so it's important to have something that's comfortable and durable.
- Exercise Clothes: Exercise clothes should be light, breathable, and stretchy. Sweatpants or leggings are great options.
- Comfortable Shoes: While Pilates can be done without shoes, investing in a comfortable pair of sneakers is highly recommended, especially if you will be doing Pilates on a regular basis.

If you want to get the most out of your Pilates sessions, make sure you take the time to warm up your muscles and joints before each session. Always be aware of your body, and listen to its feedback during and after the exercise. Make sure to work within your range of abilities, and don't overexert yourself. If you feel any discomfort, make sure to stop immediately. Finally, practice good breathing technique throughout your session to get the best results from each exercise. With proper practice, you can soon start seeing the benefits of Pilates.

PILATES MOVEMENTS

So far, we've discussed so many incredible things about wall Pilates. The magic of this type of exercise is incredible. The power and independence that you can gain are insatiable. With the strength that you build with this program, your day-to-day chores and errands will become easy again. You'll feel fresher, stronger and more stable.

The most basic wall Pilates poses are those that involve pressing your body into the wall and pushing out against the wall to work your muscles. This includes wall squats, wall push-ups, wall planks, and wall crunches.

More advanced wall Pilates poses involve moving the body in relation to the wall and using the wall as support. These poses include the wall press, where you stand a few feet away from the wall and press your palms or fists into the wall while extending your arms outwards; the wall lunge, which involves placing one foot on the wall and lunging forward with the other; and the hip extension, which involves standing perpendicular to the wall and placing your hands on the wall for support as you extend one leg behind you.

Whether you're performing basic wall Pilates exercises or advanced, your form and body alignment are the very important. This is especially true when it comes to wall pilates. Having the right posture and alignment will help you get the most out of your workout, while helping to avoid any potential injuries.

In order to ensure proper form while doing wall pilates poses, it's important to focus on keeping your core muscles engaged and your spine straight. When it comes to standing poses, your feet should be planted firmly on the floor and your hips should remain neutral. You should be aware of any tension in your body, and adjust your posture as needed. Additionally, make sure that you're breathing deeply and evenly throughout your movements.

The benefits of having proper form while doing wall pilates can include improved posture, greater flexibility and better balance. However, we'll talk more about this later in this book.

BODY ALIGNMENT

It is important to understand the body alignment and positioning when performing Pilates exercises, as it helps to maximize the benefits of the exercise and minimize the risk of injury. In this chapter, we will explore the fundamentals of body alignment during Pilates, so you can get the most out of your practice.

WHAT IS BODY ALIGNMENT?

Body alignment is the way your body is positioned relative to itself, its environment, and other objects. It is an important concept in Pilates, as proper alignment helps to promote healthy movements and avoid injury. The principles of alignment are based on the idea that the body should be symmetrical, balanced, and well-aligned when performing movements. This means that the spine should remain neutral and the shoulders, hips, knees, and feet should all be in line with one another. Proper body alignment helps to ensure that the body can move efficiently and comfortably, while also preventing injuries.

The body has several anatomical landmarks that can be used to check for proper body alignment. These include the midline of the

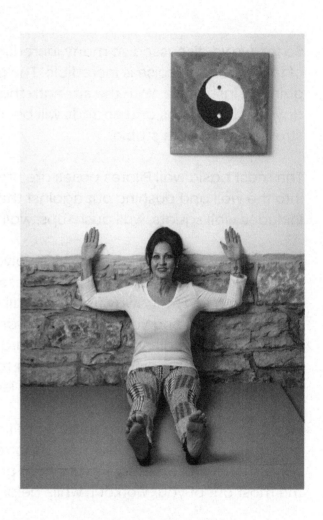

body, shoulder blades, spine, pelvis, hip joints, knees, and ankles. The body should be aligned so that these points form straight lines. Additionally, there should be equal weight distribution on both feet, and the feet should be in line with the knee. When standing in neutral position, the head should be directly over the spine, rather than jutting forward or backward.

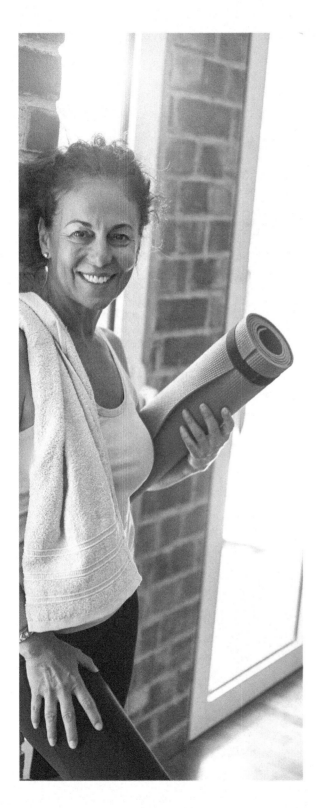

The basics of body alignment
Alignment is a key part of any Pilates practice, and it's essential for achieving maximum benefit from the exercises. Good body alignment is all about finding the right balance between being relaxed and still having control over your body.

The most important thing to understand is that the way your body moves should be directed by the core muscles. Your core muscles, located in the abdominal area, act as stabilizers and help maintain proper posture throughout your workout.

Achieving proper body alignment requires a few simple steps. First, check in with your spine – it should be straight and long. When lying down, your neck should be in line with the rest of your spine. When standing, keep your chin level with the floor and your shoulders back and relaxed.

It's also important to engage your core muscles throughout your workout. This will help you keep a good posture and protect your back from injury. Focus on squeezing your abdominal muscles inward and imagine that you are pulling your belly button towards your spine. This will engage your core muscles and support your spine throughout the workout.

Finally, it's important to keep a neutral pelvic position. This means that your hips should be level, with your tailbone pointing down towards the ground. This helps you maintain balance during the exercises and ensures that you're using the correct muscles for each move.

Remember, achieving proper body alignment takes practice, but it's worth the effort. Not only does proper alignment help you get the most out of each exercise, but it can also prevent injuries and help you achieve better overall results in your Pilates practice.

DANGERS OF POOR BODY ALIGNMENT DURING PILATES

The improper body alignment during Pilates can lead to a variety of issues including injuries, joint pains, and overworking of certain muscles. Poor body alignment can also cause muscle imbalances that can lead to more serious problems such as muscle tears and strains. Additionally, when the body is misaligned, it can lead to a decrease in posture, flexibility, and stability. This can ultimately lead to a decrease in the efficiency of your Pilates practice.

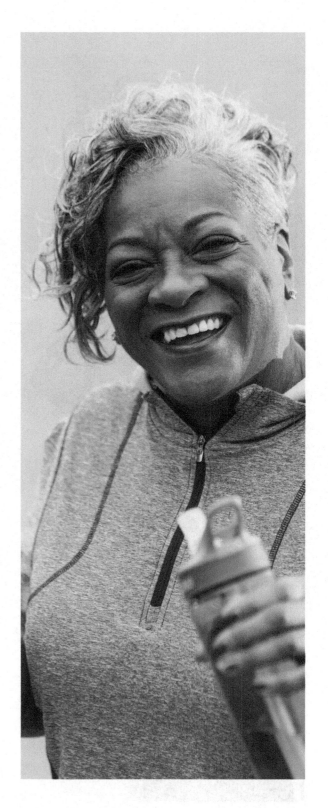

Here are some common mistakes to avoid when it comes to body alignment:

- Bending or arching the back too far
- Hyper-extending joints
- Locking out joints
- Not engaging the core muscles properly
- Not using the breath properly

If you're not sure if you're maintaining the correct body alignment during your Pilates practice, it's important to ask for help from a trained professional. They can help ensure that you're performing each exercise correctly and safely, while still getting the most out of your practice.

TIPS FOR IMPROVING YOUR BODY ALIGNMENT

START WITH A STRONG FOUNDATION

Always begin your Pilates session by paying attention to your body's foundation, starting from your feet up. Take time to make sure that your feet are firmly planted on the floor and your ankles, hips, and shoulders are all in alignment.

ENGAGE YOUR CORE MUSCLES

Pay close attention to your core muscles and keep them engaged throughout the session. This will help ensure your body is properly aligned and will also increase the intensity of your workout.

DON'T FORGET TO BREATHE

Proper breathing is key to helping you maintain the correct body alignment. Make sure to take deep breaths that fill your lungs and push out your stomach as you inhale, and then relax your abdominal muscles as you exhale.

KEEP YOUR HEAD IN LINE

The position of your head can have an effect on your body alignment. Make sure to keep your neck in line with your spine and try to avoid hunching your shoulders or jutting out your chin.

BE MINDFUL OF POSTURE

Throughout each exercise, focus on keeping the rest of your body in alignment as well. This includes keeping your shoulders back, chest lifted, and spine lengthened, as well as avoiding any excessive arching or rounding in the lower back.

By following these tips and practicing proper body alignment during Pilates, you'll be able to get the most out of every session and achieve better results in the long run.

THE IMPORTANCE OF CONTROL

One of the key elements of a successful Pilates practice is the use of controlled movements. When done correctly, these controlled movements can help maximize the benefits of Pilates and reduce the risk of injury. In this chapter, we'll discuss the importance of controlled movements in Pilates, and how they can help you get the most out of your practice.

WHY IS IT SO IMPORTANT?

A key element to any Pilates practice is executing controlled movements. Controlled movements are essential to getting the most out of Pilates because they ensure that the body is being moved in a way that works all the muscle groups involved, rather than just one or two. They also help to engage the deeper muscles which can provide more stability and protection for the joints and spine. Controlled movements also help with the coordination of movement, balance and alignment, which are all important components of Pilates. Finally, controlled movements can help to improve the mind-body connection, allowing practitioners to get the most out of their practice. In summary, controlled movements are essential to getting the most out of a Pilates practice as they help to build strength, improve alignment and enhance the mind-body connection.

HOW TO EXECUTE CONTROLLED MOVEMENTS

One of the key components of Pilates is executing controlled movements. Control is essential for proper alignment and form, which are vital to prevent injury and maximize effectiveness. Here are some tips for executing controlled movements during a Pilates workout:

FOCUS ON YOUR BREATH

As you move through each exercise, focus on inhaling and exhaling in a slow and steady rhythm. This will help keep your body relaxed and maintain good form throughout the movement.

ENGAGE YOUR CORE

Make sure that your core muscles are engaged as you move through each exercise. This helps ensure proper alignment and stability, which will lead to more effective movements.

KEEP IT SLOW AND DELIBERATE

Move slowly and deliberately as you perform each exercise. Moving too quickly can throw off your form and cause injury.

PAY ATTENTION TO YOUR FORM

Make sure that your form is correct throughout each exercise. Check your posture periodically and make corrections as needed.

USE PROPS

Utilizing props, such as yoga blocks, straps, or balls can help you achieve better alignment and control during your exercises.

Following these tips will help you execute controlled movements during your Pilates workouts, allowing you to maximize the benefits of each exercise. With regular practice, you'll find yourself achieving better form and improved control over time.

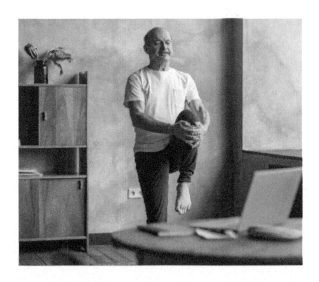

EXERCISES TO TRY TO PRACTICE CONTROL

When it comes to practicing control in Pilates, there are a few specific exercises that can help you to achieve this. Here's a few to try:

WALL CRUNCH

Wall crunches are a bodyweight exercise that is designed to help build core strength and tone the abdominal muscles. It involves leaning against a wall with your back and then crunching your torso down and up to the starting position. The crunch is an effective exercise for core stability, as it requires your abdominal muscles to work together in order to lift your body from the wall.

STANDING MOUNTAIN CLIMBERS

Standing mountain climbers are an excellent way to build core strength, increase cardiovascular endurance, and tone the muscles in your legs, arms, and torso. This full body workout involves pushing your body up and down as if you are climbing an imaginary mountain. It is easy to learn and requires no additional equipment other than your own bodyweight. With this exercise, you will gain more mobility, flexibility, and power. Regular standing mountain climbers will help you gain strength and become a more agile climber.

KNEE TO CHEST
Knee to chest exercises are an effective way to strengthen your core and lower back muscles. This exercise involves standing on your feet with one knee bent and then bringing one knee up towards your chest at a time. As you raise your knee, you can either use your hands to gently pull it towards your chest or press it into your hands as you squeeze your core muscles. This simple exercise can help you build strength and flexibility in your core and lower back.

SEATED ACTIVE FORWARD FOLD
Seated Active Forward Fold is a seated stretching pose that increases flexibility and helps to ease tension. The pose involves bending the body forward while seated with the legs straight in front. The spine is arched slightly and the arms are kept straight out. This pose strengthens and stretches the legs, core, back and arms while promoting balance, stability, and increased flexibility. Additionally, Seated Active Forward Fold helps to calm the mind, relieving anxiety and fatigue.

"You are never too old to make fitness a part of your life - no matter your age, movement is the key to longevity and happiness."

THE WALL PILATES PROGRAM

Our wall Pilates program is very flexible and allows you to build on strength at your own pace. You don't have to perform advanced poses straight away to feel results. It's all about you and your current level. Be patient and be committed. Start with the daily gentle routine, and if you feel good, then move on to the next stage (and so on). Take your time and remember what we discussed throughout this book.

To begin with, depending on how you;re feeling, maybe start with one routine a week and then performing the following routines the weeks after. Increase how often you're performing then with a goal in mind to train for 28 days. So, it's all about building your strength gradually and helping you build enough strength that you can train for 28 days without pain or strain. In addition to building up your resilience, remember to stop 15-20 seconds between each exercise to give yourself time to rest. Overworking yourself can be bad for your heart, so make sure to do each routine at your own pace.

Lastly, before we dive into the poses and exercises. It's important that you stretch before and after each routine. Stretching before and after exercise is an important part of any exercise routine. Stretching helps increase range of motion in your muscles, improves your overall flexibility, and reduces your risk of injury. Additionally, stretching helps to relax and reduce muscle tension, so that your body is better able to perform during exercise and recover afterward.

Before you begin an exercise routine, stretching can help your muscles prepare for the activity to come. A short stretching routine can help increase blood flow to your muscles, and helps increase flexibility and range of motion. This means that when you do exercise, you'll be able to work with a wider range of motion and a greater range of motion. Additionally, when you stretch before a workout, you can help reduce any muscle soreness and help prepare your body for the exercise you're about to do.

After exercise, stretching can help your body relax and reduce muscle tension. After a workout, stretching can help you increase the blood flow to your muscles and reduce muscle soreness. It also helps to improve your posture and reduce the risk of injury due to muscle tension. Additionally, stretching after exercise can help you speed up the process of recovery and return to a state of normal functioning quicker. Here's 5 top stretches you can use:

SHOULDER SHRUGS
To start, stand straight and lift your shoulders up to your ears. Hold this for five seconds, then relax. Repeat 10 times.

SIDE BENDS
To do this stretch, stand straight with feet hip width apart. Keep your shoulders and neck relaxed and arms to the side. Bend your torso to the left and hold for 5 seconds. Then, do the same on the other side.

NECK ROLLS
Sitting comfortably in a chair, gently lower your chin towards your chest. From there, move your head in a circular motion. Slowly roll your head forward and then backward in a clockwise and counter-clockwise direction. Make sure you roll the head back in one slow continuous motion.

CALF STRETCH
To stretch the calf muscle, stand at arm's length from a wall and place your right foot in front of the other. Step forward and place your right hand against the wall. Bend your right knee and press your heel into the ground as you straighten the other leg. Hold the stretch for 20-30 seconds and repeat with the left leg.

STANDING HAMSTRING STRETCH
This stretch requires a sturdy chair. Begin by standing behind the chair, hold on with your hands, and bend your torso forward until you can feel the stretch in the back of your thigh. Hold for 10-15 seconds, then return to a standing position. Repeat for the other side.

WALL PILATES ROUTINES

DAILY GENTLE ROUTINE (10 MINS)

Seated Active Forward Fold

Seated Knee to Chest

Opposite Toe Reach

Seated Arm Mobility

Active Frog Stretch

Single leg Series (left)

Single leg Series (Right)

Lying Walks to Bridge

Reach Through Crunch

Wall Crunch

POSTURE AND CORE ROUTINE (10 MINS)

Supported Side Bends

Shoulder Press

Wall Supported Waiter

Standing Mountain Climbers

Knee to chest (left)

Knee to chest (right)

Reach Through Crunch

Crunch Pulses

MAGIC BALANCE ROUTINE (15 MINS)

- Triceps Wall Push-ups
- Robot Arms
- Chest Wall Push Ups
- Chest Opener
- Wall Arm Press Hold (Palms to the front)
- Wall Arm Press Hold (Palms to the wall)
- Wall Supported Bird Dog (Left Arm)
- Wall Supported Bird Dog (Right Arm)
- Supported Semi Lunge (Left)
- Supported Semi Lunge (Right)
- Wall sits
- Double Knee Bends
- Butterfly Openers
- Alternating Side Hip Slides
- Alternating Leg Abduction

FLEXIBILITY & ABS ENANCHEMENT ROUTINE (17 MINS)

- Supported Side Bends
- Upper Back Roll
- Wall Side Bends (Left)
- Wall Side Bends (Right)
- Supported Roll Down
- Standing Mountain Climbers
- Seated Active Forward Fold
- Seated Opposite Toe Reach
- Supported Spine Twist
- Wall Crunch
- Side To Side Crunch
- Reach Through Crunch
- Knee to Chest (Right)
- Lifted knee to Chest (Right)
- Knee to Chest (Left)
- Lifted Knee to Chest (Left)
- Tabletop Oblique Twist

EXERCISE INSTRUCTIONS

SEATED ACTIVE FORWARD FOLD (60 SEC)

This exercise stretches your hamstrings and calve muscles. It will mobilize your lower and upper back.

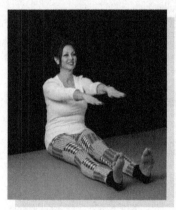 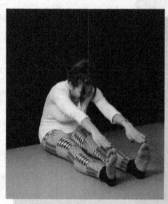

COMMON MISTAKES TO AVOID

- Reducing range of motion
- Bending the arms or legs

GENERAL TIPS:

- Breathe steadily throughout the exercise.
- Maintain a straight back and avoid rounding your spine.

INSTRUCTIONS:

1. Sit against a wall with your legs extended in front of you.
2. Extend your arms up towards the ceiling, keeping them straight and parallel to each other.
3. Straddle your legs wider than hip width apart.
4. Slowly bend forward at the hips, reaching your hands towards your toes.
5. Hold the position for a few seconds, then slowly return to the starting position.

SEATED KNEE TO CHEST (60 SEC)

The Seated Knee to Chest exercise is great for activating your hip flexor muscles.

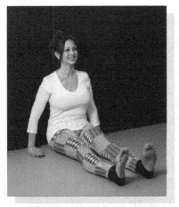
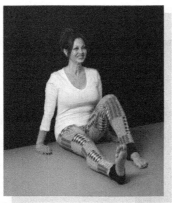
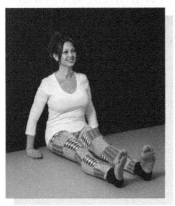
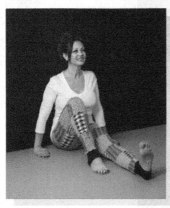

INSTRUCTIONS:

1. Sit against a wall with your back straight.
2. Keep your hands next to your sides and your legs straight.
3. Without lifting your leg, slide one knee up towards your chest.
4. Return your leg to the starting position and repeat on the other side.

COMMON MISTAKES TO AVOID

- Only doing one side.
- Arching your lower back

GENERAL TIPS:

- Remember to maintain a steady breathing pattern while doing this exercise.

SEATED OPPOSITE TOE REACH (60 SEC)

This exercise stretches your spinal erector muscles and your hamstrings and calves.

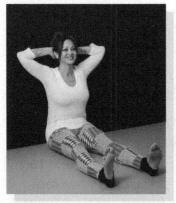 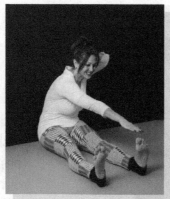

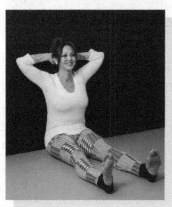 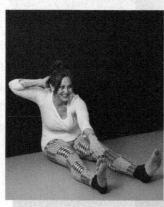

INSTRUCTIONS:

1. Sit tall against a wall with legs straddled.
2. Bend arms behind your head.
3. Reach with your left hand towards your right toes.
4. Keep your right arm bent behind your head.
5. Return to starting position.
6. Repeat on the other side.

COMMON MISTAKES TO AVOID

- Doing one side only
- Bending the knees
- Holding your breath

GENERAL TIPS:

- Inhale at the beginning of the movement and exhale slowly as you reach towards your toes.
- Maintain a steady breathing pattern throughout the exercise.

SEATED ARM MOBILITY (60 SEC)

This exercise improves your internal and external shoulder mobility and is an excellent warm up choice.

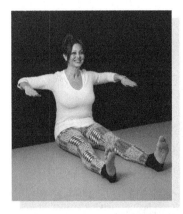
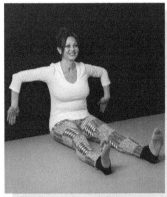
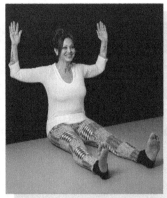
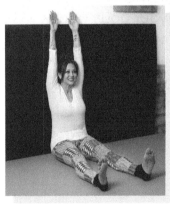
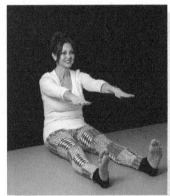
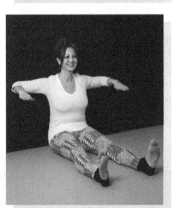

COMMON MISTAKES TO AVOID

- Going too fast: Perform the movement slowly and with control.
- Arc hing the lower back: Keep your back straight and avoid overarching.

GENERAL TIPS:

- Maintain a steady breathing pattern throughout the exercise.
- Use a cushion for support if needed.

INSTRUCTIONS:

1. Sit tall against a wall.
2. Extend arms forward
3. Keep your legs straddled.
4. Bend your elbows backwards at 90-degrees angle.
5. When your elbows touch the wall, rotate your hands down to the wall.
6. From there, rotate them up and glide arms up.

ACTIVE FROG STRETCH (60 SEC)

This dynamic stretch targets the adductor muscles and improves hip mobility. It is a great warm up exercise for squats.

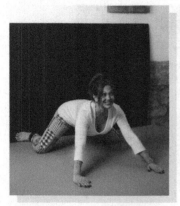
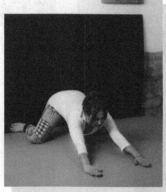
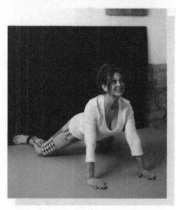

INSTRUCTIONS:

1. Start on the floor, resting on your hands.
2. Open your knees as wide as possible and put your feet on the wall.
3. Rock your body backward and forward.
4. Keep your lower back straight.

COMMON MISTAKES TO AVOID

- Arching the lower back: Keep your back straight and avoid overarching.
- Not keeping the knees wide enough: Open your knees as wide as possible to target the adductor muscles effectively.

GENERAL TIPS:

- Maintain a steady breathing pattern throughout the exercise.

SINGLE LEG SERIES (LEFT) (60 SEC)

This exercise is an excellent choice for dynamically opening your hips and stretching your adductor muscles. It's best to perform it before engaging in heavy lower body exercises. Follow these instructions to do it properly.

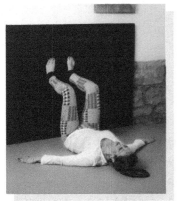
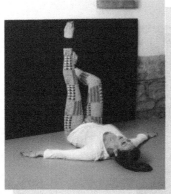
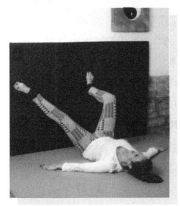
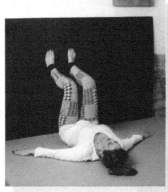

INSTRUCTIONS:

1. Lie flat on your back.
2. Place your knees against the wall at a 90 degree angle.
3. Ex tend your left leg up and slowly bring it down to your left side without moving your pelvis.
4. Return your leg to the starting position.
5. Repeat the exercise on the other side.

COMMON MISTAKES TO AVOID

- Bending your leg during the movement.
- Allowing your leg to fall uncontrollably to the side
- Moving your pelvis during the exercise.

GENERAL TIPS:

- Inhale at the beginning of the movement and slowly exhale as you lower your leg.
- Keep your movements slow and controlled.
- Straighten your leg to en gage your adductor muscles.

SINGLE LEG SERIES (RIGHT) (60 SEC)

This exercise is an effective way to dynamically open your hips and stretch your adductor muscles. It's highly recommended to do it before engaging in heavier lower body exercises.

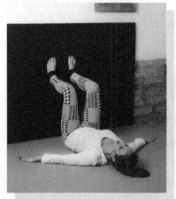 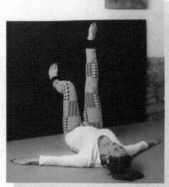

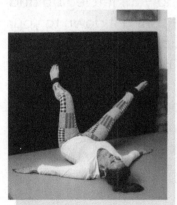 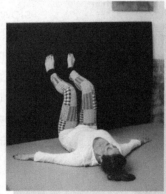

INSTRUCTIONS:

1. Lie on your back.
2. Place your knees against the wall at a 90 degree angle.
3. Lift your right leg up and bring it down to your right side, without moving your pelvis.
4. Return your leg to the starting position.
5. Repeat the exercise on your left side.

COMMON MISTAKES TO AVOID

- Bending your leg during the exercise.
- Allowing your leg to fall uncontrollably to the side.
- Moving your pelvis while performing the exercise.

GENERAL TIPS:

- Inhale at the beginning and exhale slowly.
- Keep your movements controlled.

LYING WALKS TO BRIDGE (60 SEC)

Lying walks through bridge is an effective way to activate your glutes and hamstrings. Use it as a pre activation exercise during your warm up routine.

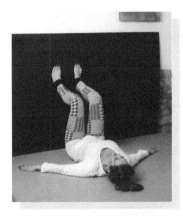
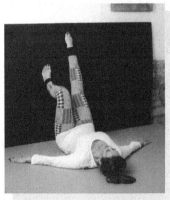
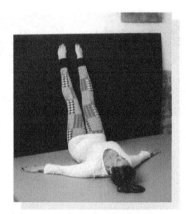
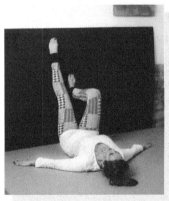
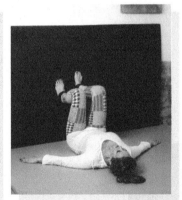
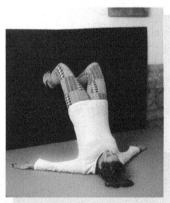

COMMON MISTAKES TO AVOID

- Holding your breath.
- Arching your lower back.
- Allowing your hips to lower uncontrollably.

GENERAL TIPS:

- For added difficulty, hold a dumbbell on your stomach.
- Remember to maintain control and breathe consistently throughout t he exercise.

INSTRUCTIONS:

1. Lie on your back with your knees bent at a 90 degree angle against a wall.
2. Lift one leg up, then the other.
3. Bring both legs back down to the starting position and push your hips up.

WALL CRUNCH (60 SEC)

Perform this effective exercise to engage your abs and stretch your back muscles.

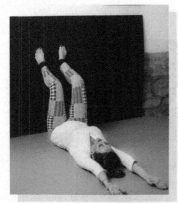
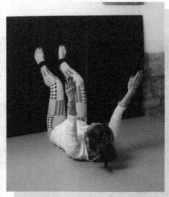

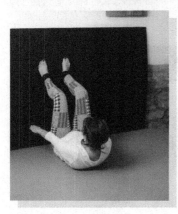

INSTRUCTIONS:

1. Lie flat on your back and place your knees at a 90 degree angle against a wall.
2. Extend your arms backwards beside your head.
3. Tighten your abs and crunch up, bringing your arms forward to touch the floor with your fingers.

COMMON MISTAKES TO AVOID

- Arching your lower back
- Failing to lift your shoulders off the floor
- Using momentum

GENERAL TIPS:

- Breathe in at the start of the movement and exhale slowly while crunching.
- This breathing technique will increase the activation of your abs.

REACH THROUGH CRUNCH (60 SEC)

Reach Through Crunch is an effective exercise for activating your abdominal muscles.

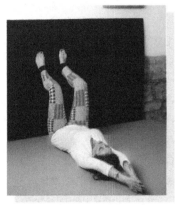 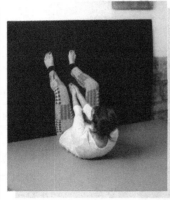

INSTRUCTIONS:

1. Lie on your back with your knees bent at a 90 degree angle against a wall.
2. Extend your arms over your head and place your hands together.
3. Engage your core and bring your hands between your knees.

COMMON MISTAKES TO AVOID

- Arching your lower back.
- Not lifting your shoulders off the floor.
- Using momentum.

GENERAL TIPS:

- Inhale at the beginning of the movement and exhale slowly as you crunch.
- Focus on performing the exercise with control and without rushing through the motion.

SUPPORTED SIDE BENDS (90 SEC)

To dynamically stretch your latissimus dorsi and external oblique abdominal muscles, try Supported Side Bends:

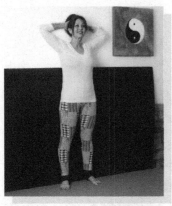
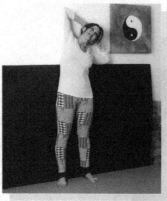
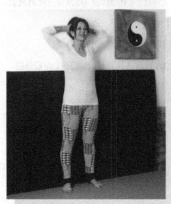
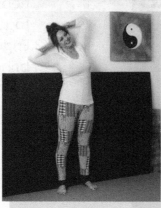

INSTRUCTIONS:

1. Stand tall with a narrower stance.
2. Pin your posterior chain to the wall.
3. Put your hands on the backside of your head.
4. Bend your body sideways and return to a standing position.
5. Do the same on both sides.

COMMON MISTAKES TO AVOID

- Holding your breath
- Doing only one side
- Moving too quickly

GENERAL TIPS:

- Inhale at the beginning of the movement, and slowly exhale as you start bending to the side.
- Exhaling engages more of your abdominal muscles.

WALL SUPPORTED WAITER (90 SEC)

Wall Shoulder Press is an excellent exercise that improves posture and strengthens your shoulders and mid back muscles.

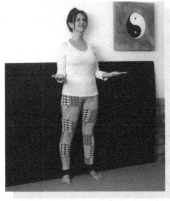
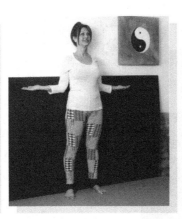

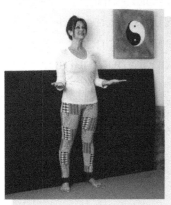

INSTRUCTIONS:

1. Stand tall against the wall.
2. Pin your glutes, head, and upper back to the wall.
3. Bend your elbows at a 90 degree angle.
4. Glide your arms up.
5. Glide your elbows down to your sides.
6. Do multiple repetitions.

COMMON MISTAKES TO AVOID

- Taking the elbows off the wall
- Holding your breath
- Moving too quickly

GENERAL TIPS:

- If you lack mobility, take one step away from the wall.
- You can gently bend your knees to flatten your back even more.

SHOULDER PRESS (90 SEC)

Wall Shoulder Press is an excellent exercise that improves posture and strengthens your shoulders and mid back muscles.

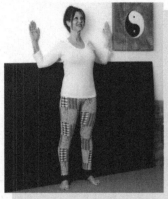 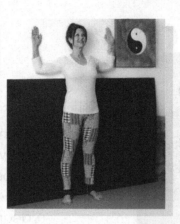

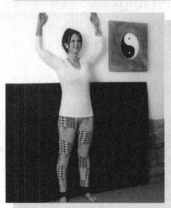

INSTRUCTIONS:

1. Stand tall against the wall.
2. Pin your glutes, head, elbows, and upper back to the wall.
3. Bring your hands forward at a 90 degree angle.
4. Move your hands to the side until your thumbs touch the wall!

COMMON MISTAKES TO AVOID

- Taking the elbows off the wall.
- Going too fast.
- Holding the breath.

GENERAL TIPS:

- To increase the intensity of the exercise, hold a light weight in each hand
- Focus on keeping your shoulders down and back throughout the movement to engage the correcmuscles.

STANDING MOUNTAIN CLIMBERS (90 SEC)

Standing Mountain Climbers are an excellent exercise for improving overall fitness levels and working the cardiovascular system.

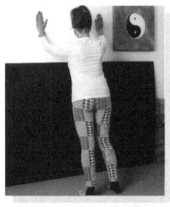
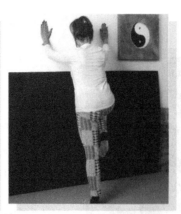
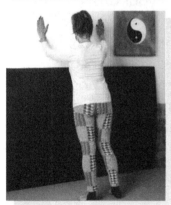
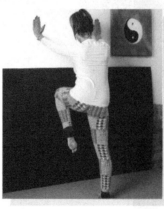

INSTRUCTIONS:

1. Stand tall with feet shoulder width apart.
2. Place your hands on the wall for support with arms extended.
3. Lift one knee up, bring it down, and then lift the other knee.
4. Keep your back straight.

COMMON MISTAKES TO AVOID

- Doing only one side
- Holding your breath

GENERAL TIPS:

- To make this exercise more intense, alternate your legs at a faster pace.

KNEE TO CHEST (LEFT) (90 SEC)

Knee to Chest is an exercise that can activate your hip flexor muscles and help build strength in that area.

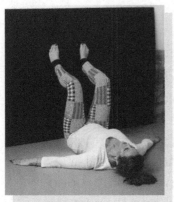 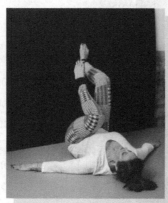

INSTRUCTIONS:

1. Lie flat on your back.
2. Place your knees at a 90 degree angle against a wall.
3. Extend your arms out to the sides.
4. Lift and bring one knee toward your chest.
5. Lower your leg back to the starting position and repeat with the other leg.

COMMON MISTAKES TO AVOID

- Moving too quickly
- Holding your breath
- Arching your lower back

GENERAL TIPS:

- Try to maintain a steady breathing pat tern throughout the exercise.
- If it's difficult, focus on exhaling as you bring your knee toward your chest.

KNEE TO CHEST (RIGHT) (60 SEC)

Knee to Chest is an exercise that can activate your hip flexor muscles and help build strength in that area.

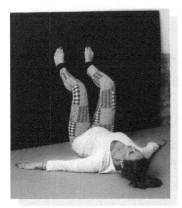 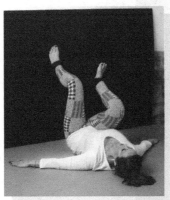

INSTRUCTIONS:

1. Lay flat on your back.
2. Put your knees at a 90 degree angle against a wall.
3. Extend your arms to your sides.
4. Lift and bring your right knee towards your chest.

COMMON MISTAKES TO AVOID

- Moving too quickly
- Holding your breath
- Arching your lower back

GENERAL TIPS:

- Focus on maintaining a steady breathing pattern throughout the exercise.
- Keep your body relax ed and your movements controlled.

WALL CRUNCH (60 SEC)

Perform this effective exercise to engage your abs and stretch your back muscles.

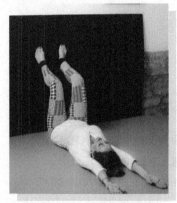
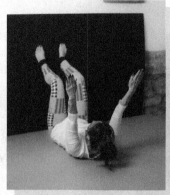
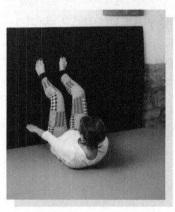

INSTRUCTIONS:

1. Lie flat on your back and place your knees at a 90 degree angle against a wall.
2. Extend your arms backwards beside your head.
3. Tighten your abs and crunch up, bringing your arms forward to touch the floor with your fingers.

COMMON MISTAKES TO AVOID

- Arching your lower back
- Failing to lift your shoulders off the floor.
- Using momentum

GENERAL TIPS:

- Breathe in at the start of the movement and exhale slowly while crunching.
- This breathing technique will increase the activation of your abs.

CRUNCH PULSES (60 SEC)

Crunch Pulses are an effective exercise that targets your abdominal muscles and can help strengthen your core.

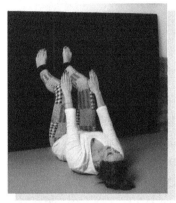
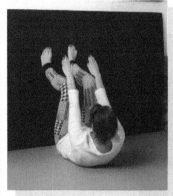
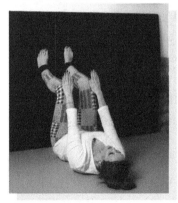
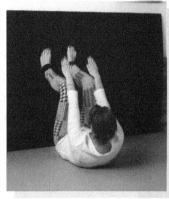

INSTRUCTIONS:

1. Lie flat on your back.
2. Bend your knees at a 90 degree angle with your feet on the wall.
3. Place your hands on your thighs.
4. Tighten your abs and lift your shoulders off the floor.
5. Let your hands travel past your knees.

COMMON MISTAKES TO AVOID

- Not lifting your shoulders off the floor
- Rushing the movemen
- Holding your breath

GENERAL TIPS:

- Inhale at the beginning of the movement and slowly exhale as you start crunching.
- Remember to maintain a steady breathing pattern throughout the exercise.

TRICEPS WALL PUSH UPS (60 SEC)

Triceps Wall Push Ups are a great exercise to develop your triceps and condition your tendons for heavier variations of push ups.

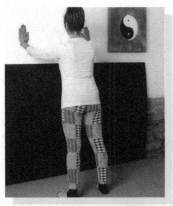 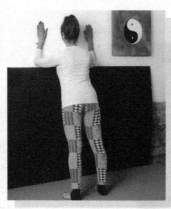

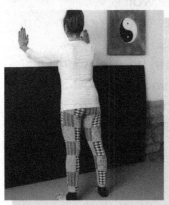

INSTRUCTIONS:

1. Stand tall with your feet slightly narrower than shoulder width apart.
2. Place your hands onto the wall at chest level with your fingers pointing upwards.
3. Keep your elbows close to your sides throughout the movement.
4. Slowly lower yourself towards the wall by bending your elbows until your chest touches the wall.
5. Push yourself back up to the starting position by straightening your elbows.

COMMON MISTAKES TO AVOID

- Allowing your elbows to flare out to the sides.
- Not lowering yourself fully to the wall
- Dropping your body instead of controlling the descent.
- Holding your breath.

GENERAL TIPS:

- Inhale deeply before starting the movement and exhale as you push yourself back up.
- Keep your core engaged and maintain a straight line from your head to your heels.

ROBOT ARMS (60 SEC)

Robot arm is an effective exercise for enhancing both internal and external shoulder mobility while strengthening your rotator cuff muscles.

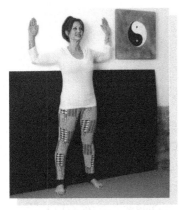 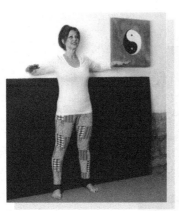

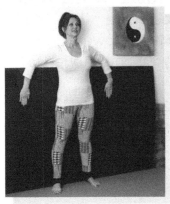

INSTRUCTIONS:

1. Stand with your back against a wall.
2. Place your elbows on the wall at a 90 degree angle, with the back of your palms touching the wall.
3. Slowly rotate your arms down until the front of your palms touch the wall, then return to the starting position.

COMMON MISTAKES TO AVOID

- Rushing through the exercise too quickly.
- Lifting your elbows away from the wall.

GENERAL TIPS:

- To add resistance and make the exercise more challenging, try using light wrist weights.
- Focus on maintaining control throughout the movement.

CHEST WALL PUSH UPS (60 SEC)

Chest Wall Push Up is a great exercise that targets your chest and triceps muscles and helps to condition your tendons for heavier variations of push ups

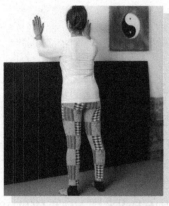
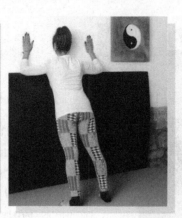
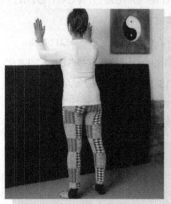

INSTRUCTIONS:

1. Stand tall with your feet a bit narrower.
2. Put your hands onto the wall at your chest level.
3. Keep your elbows at a 45 degree angle.
4. From there, lower yourself until your chest touches the wall.
5. Push yourself up.

COMMON MISTAKES TO AVOID

- Not keeping your elbows at a 45 degree angle.
- Partial range of motion.
- Holding your breath.

GENERAL TIPS:

- Inhale at the beginning of the movement, and slowly exhale as you push yourself up.
- Always keep your elbows at a 45 degree angle.

CHEST OPENERS (60 SEC)

Chest Openers, as the name itself suggests, activate your pectoral muscles and are great for improving posture.

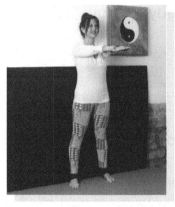 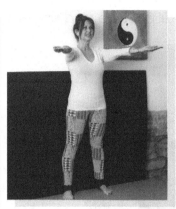

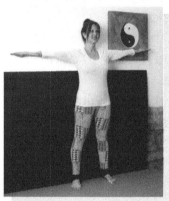

INSTRUCTIONS:

1. Stand tall with a narrow stance.
2. Pin your posterior chain (backside of your body) to the wall.
3. Extend your arms at a 90 degree angle.
4. Rotate your palms towards the ceiling.
5. From there, bring your hands together

COMMON MISTAKES TO AVOID

- Moving your body away from the wall
- Holding your breath.
- Going too fast.

GENERAL TIPS:

- Maintain a steady breathing pattern throughout the exercise to reduce tension
- Focus on squeezing your shoulder blades together to get a deeper stretch in your chest muscles.

WALL ARM PRESS HOLD(60 SEC)

This exercise will activate your mid back, deltoid, and triceps muscles, making it an excellent way to improve your posture and upper body strength.

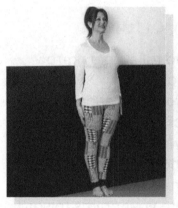 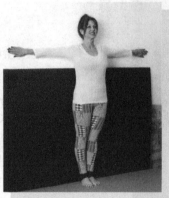

INSTRUCTIONS:

1. Stand tall against the wall.
2. Pin your glutes, head, and upper back to the wall.
3. Keep your arms next to your sides.
4. From there, lift your arms sideways to a 90 degree angle.
5. Press the wall with your palms facing the wall.
6. Hold this position for a few seconds.

COMMON MISTAKES TO AVOID

- Bending the arms.
- Holding your breath.
- Not holding the static position.

GENERAL TIPS:

- Inhale at the beginning of the movement and slowly exhale as you start pressing your palms against the wall.
- Focus on keeping your shoulders down and your neck relaxed throughout the exercise.

SUPPORTED SEMI LUNGE (LEFT) (60 SEC)

The following exercise will help strengthen your legs, especially if you're dealing with strength imbalances.

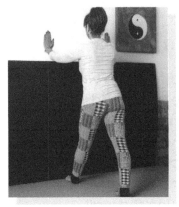 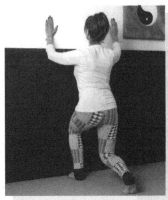

INSTRUCTIONS:

1. Stand facing a wall and place your hands on the wall at shoulder height.
2. Step your left foot forward and bring your toes close to the wall.
3. Step your rig ht foot back, maintaining a comfortable distance between your fee.
4. Keeping your torso upright, bend both knees to a 45 degree angle by leaning forward.

COMMON MISTAKES TO AVOID

- Going too low, which can strain your knees and back.
- Holding your breath, which can affect your performance and increase tension in your body.
- Rushing the movement, which can compromise your form and reduce its effectiveness.

GENERAL TIPS:

- Inhale at the start of the movement and exhale slowly as you continue bending your knees.
- Maintain a steady breathing pattern throughout the exercise.

SUPPORTED SEMI LUNGE (RIGHT) (60 SEC)

This exercise will strengthen your legs. It is great to do if you are dealing with some strength imbalances n your legs.

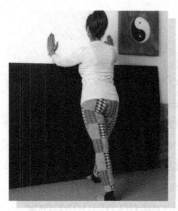 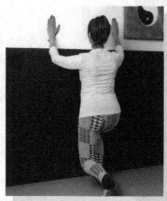

INSTRUCTIONS:

1. Stand facing a wall and place your hands on the wall at shoulder height.
2. Step your right foot forward and place it flat on the ground with your toes touching the wall.
3. Step your left foot back, keeping your heel off the ground.
4. Bend both knees to 45 degrees by leaning forward slightly, keeping your torso straight and your hips level.
5. Hold the lunge for a few seconds before returning to the starting position.

COMMON MISTAKES TO AVOID

- Going too low, which can strain your knees.
- Holding your breath, which can make the exercise harder.
- Rushing the movement, which can compromise form and effectiveness.

GENERAL TIPS:

- Inhale as you start to bend your knees and exhale as you rise back up.
- Keep your core engaged and your chest up throughout the movement.
- If you have trouble balancing, try placing your hands on a sturdy chair instead of the wa ll.

WALL SIT (60 SEC)

Supported Semi Squat is a phenomenal exercise that will strengthen your quadriceps and glute muscles, as well as your quadriceps tendon.

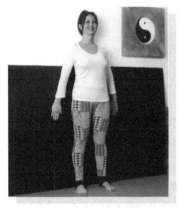
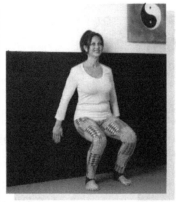
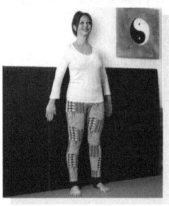

INSTRUCTIONS:

1. Stand tall with your feet about one step away from the wall.
2. Pin your head, back, and glutes against the wall.
3. Slide down until your knees reach a 45 degree angle.
4. Hold the static stretch.
5. Slowly rise back up.

COMMON MISTAKES TO AVOID

- Going too low or not bending your knees enough.
- Holding your breath.
- Not keeping your posterior chain pinned to the wall.

GENERAL TIPS:

- Focus on keeping your knees aligned with your toes and avoid letting them cave i n.
- Breathe deeply throughout the exercise to maximize oxygen flow to your muscles.

DOUBLE KNEE BENDS (60 SEC)

This exercise is great for dynamically stretching your latissimus dorsi muscle while also activating your hamstrings and hip flexors.

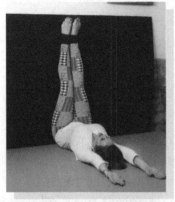
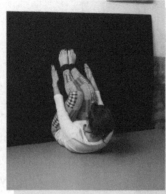
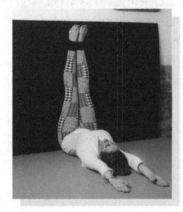

INSTRUCTIONS:

1. Lie flat on your back.
2. Extend your knees onto the wall.
3. Engage your abdominals.
4. Extend your arms next to your head.
5. Slowly slide your feet down while bringing your elbows towards your knees.
6. Return to the starting position.

COMMON MISTAKES TO AVOID

- Arching the back
- Not engaging the abdominals

GENERAL TIPS:

- Remember to inhale at the beginning of the movement and slowly exhale as you bring your arms forward.

BUTTERFLY OPENERS (60 SEC)

Butterfly Openers are a great exercise that targets external hip rotation and activates the pectoral muscles.

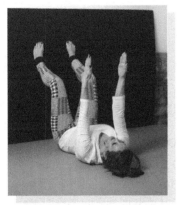
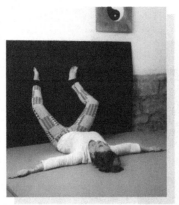
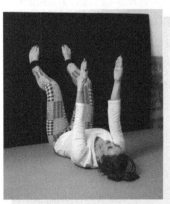

INSTRUCTIONS:

1. Lie flat on your back with your arms extended upright.
2. Place your feet on the wall and bend your knees to a 90 degree angle.
3. Open your knees and arms simultaneously.
4. Briig your knees and arms back together.

COMMON MISTAKES TO AVOID

- Rushing the movement
- Arching the back
- Holding the breath.

GENERAL TIPS:

- Inhale at the beginning of the movement and exhale slowly as you open your legs and arms.
- Keep your back flat on the ground throughout the exercise.

ALTERNATING SIDE HIP SIDES (60 SEC)

Alternating Side Hip Slides are an excellent exercise that targets your pectoral muscles and improves external hip mobility, while also stretching your adductor muscles.

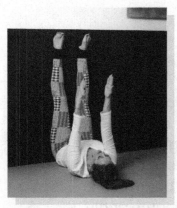
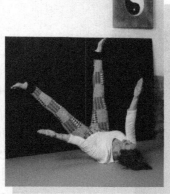

INSTRUCTIONS:

1. Lie flat on your back.
2. Keep your legs extended up the wall.
3. Extend your arms upright.
4. Simultaneously bring your left leg and left arm down.
5. Go back up, and then do the same on the other side.

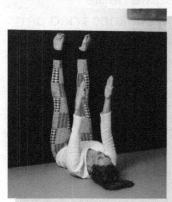
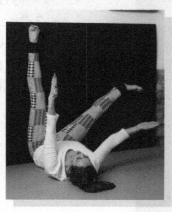

COMMON MISTAKES TO AVOID

- Letting your pelvis move around.
- Arching your lower back.
- Holding your breath.

GENERAL TIPS:

- To make sure your pelvis remains stable, focus on pushing your bellybutton towards the floor.
- Remember to breathe throughout the exercise.

ALTERNATING LEG ABDUCTION (60 SEC)

Alternating Leg Abduction is a great exercise to improve your hip mobility and stretch your adductor muscles.

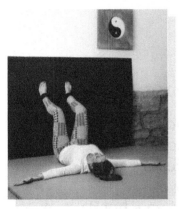
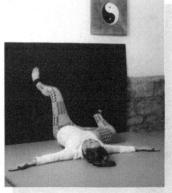
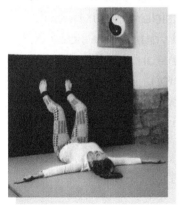
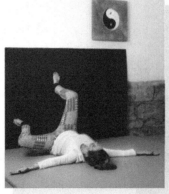

INSTRUCTIONS:

1. Lie flat on the floor with your arms extended next to your sides.
2. Place your feet on the wall, maintaining a 90 degree angle at the knees.
3. Slide one foot down to the side while keeping your pelvis on the floor.
4. Return the foot to the starting position and repeat with the other leg.

COMMON MISTAKES TO AVOID

- Arching the lower back
- Letting your pelvis move off the floor
- Doing the exercise only on one side

GENERAL TIPS:

- To prevent your pelvis from moving off the floor, think about pushing your belly button to the floor.
- Keep the movement controlled and avoid rushed movements.

SUPPORTED SIDE BENDS (60 SEC)

Supported Side Bends are an effective exercise to dynamically stretch your latissimus dorsi and external oblique abdominal muscles.

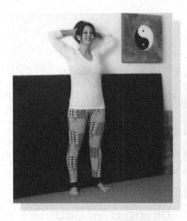
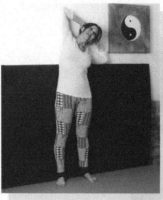
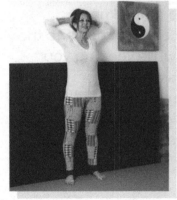
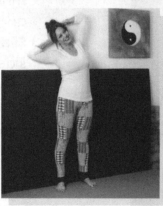

INSTRUCTIONS:

1. Stand tall with a narrow stance.
2. Pin your posterior chain to the wall.
3. Place your hands on the backside of your head.
4. Bend your body sideways and return to the starting position.
5. Repeat on both sides.

COMMON MISTAKES TO AVOID

- Holding your breath
- Only performing the exercise on one si d
- Moving too quickly

GENERAL TIPS:

- Remember to inhale at the start of the movement and exhale slowly as you bend to the side.

UPPER BACK ROLL (60 SEC)

This exercise is designed to stretch your neck and upper back muscles. It's particularly beneficial if you're experiencing stiffness in these areas.

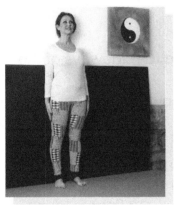 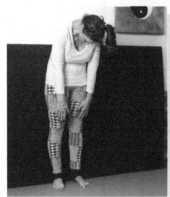

INSTRUCTIONS:

1. Stand with your feet close together.
2. Press your head, upper back, and glutes against the wall.
3. Keep your knees straight.
4. Roll your head and upper back forward to round your spine.
5. Stop when your upper back is rounded, then return to the starting position and repeat the movement.

COMMON MISTAKES TO AVOID

- Rounding your spine excessively.
- Bending your knees
- Holding your breath.

GENERAL TIPS:

- Inhale at the beginning of the movement and exhale slowly as you round your upper back.

WALL SIDE BENDS (LEFT) (60 SEC)

This exercise is great for stretching your neck and upper back muscles, especially if you're feeling stiff in those areas.

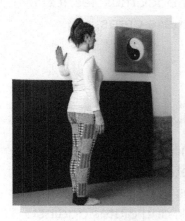
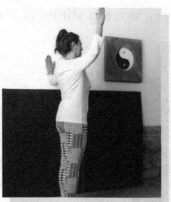
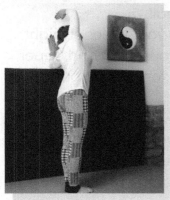

INSTRUCTIONS:

1. Stand tall sideways of the wall.
2. Put your left hand onto the wall.
3. Bend towards your left side while lifting your right arm up and above your head.
4. When your fingers touch together return to previous position.

COMMON MISTAKES TO AVOID

- Rounding your back more than is recommended.
- Bending your knees.
- Holding your breath.

GENERAL TIPS:

- Remember to inhale at the beginning of the movement and exhale slowly as you round your upper back.

WALL SIDE BENDS (RIGHT) (60 SEC)

Wall Side Bends are a great exercise for stretching your latissimus dorsi muscle and external oblique abdominal muscles.

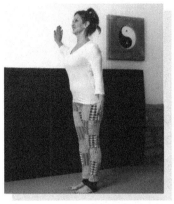
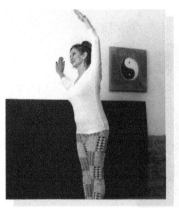
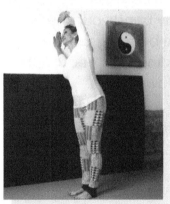

INSTRUCTIONS:

1. Stand tall sideways of the wall.
2. Put your right hand onto the wall.
3. Bend towards your right side while lifting your left arm up and above your head.
4. When your fingers touch together return to previous position.

COMMON MISTAKES TO AVOID

- Bending the arms.
- Bending the legs
- Arching your lower back.

GENERAL TIPS:

- If you can't touch your fingers together, don't worry, just go as far as you can while maintaining comfort.

SUPPORTED ROLL DOWN (60 SEC)

Supported Roll downs are a fantastic way to stretch your upper and lower back, as well as your hamstrings.

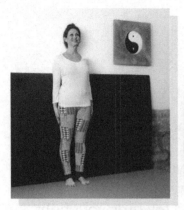
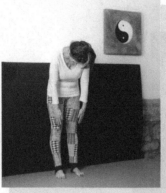
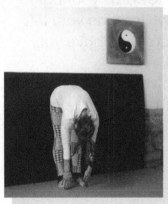

INSTRUCTIONS:

1. Stand with your feet narrow.
2. Place your head, upper back, and glutes against the wall.
3. Gently bend your knees.
4. Begin bending forward by rounding your head, upper and lower back.
5. Allow your arms to relax towards the floor.

COMMON MISTAKES TO AVOID

- Bending the knees too much.
- Holding your breath.
- Not keeping your glutes against the wall.

GENERAL TIPS:

- Inhale at the beginning of the movement, and slowly exhale as you start folding forward.

STANDING MOUNTAIN CLIMBERS (60 SEC)

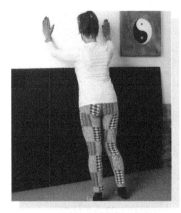
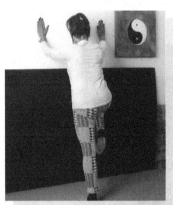
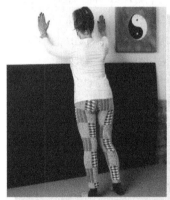
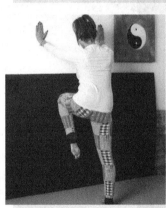

INSTRUCTIONS:

1. Stand tall with your feet shoulder width apart.
2. Place your hands on a wall to support yourself.
3. Keep your arms extended.
4. Lift one knee up towards your chest, then lower it back down.
5. Immediately lift the other knee up towards your chest, then lower it back down.
6. Continue alternating legs in a quick, rhythmic motion.
7. Keep your back straight and engaged throughout the movement.

COMMON MISTAKES TO AVOID

- Only performing the exercise on one side.
- Holding your breath.

GENERAL TIPS:

- To increase the intensity of the exercise, try performing it at a faster pace.
- Keep your core engaged throughout the exercise for added stability.

SEATED ACTIVE FORWARD FOLD (60 SEC)

This exercise stretches your hamstrings and calve muscles. It will mobilize your lower and upper back.

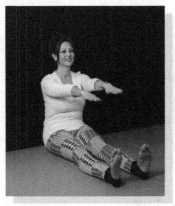 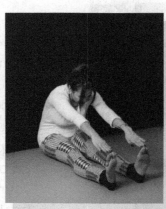

INSTRUCTIONS:

1. Sit against a wall with your legs extended in front of you.
2. Extend your arms up towards the ceiling, keeping them straight and parallel to each other.
3. Straddle your legs wider than hip width apart.
4. Slowly bend forward at the hips, reaching your hands towards your toes.
5. Hold the position for a few seconds, then slowly return to the starting position.

COMMON MISTAKES TO AVOID

- Reducing range of motion
- Bending the arms or legs

GENERAL TIPS:

- Breathe steadily throughout the exercise.
- Maintain a straight back and avoid rounding your spine.

SEATED OPPOSITE TOE REACH (60 SEC)

This exercise stretches your spinal erector muscles and also your hamstrings and calves.

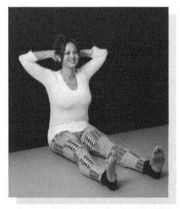
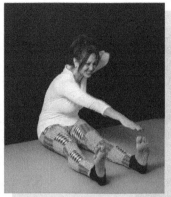
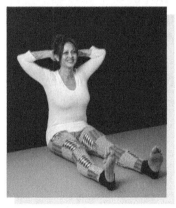
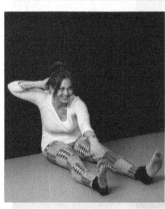

INSTRUCTIONS:

1. Sit tall against a wall with legs straddled.
2. Bend arms behind your head.
3. Reach with your left hand towards your right toes.
4. Keep your right arm bent behind your head.
5. Return to starting position.
6. Repeat on the other side.

COMMON MISTAKES TO AVOID

- Doing one side only.
- Bending the knees
- Holding your breath.

GENERAL TIPS:

- Inhale at the beginning of the movement and exhale slowly as you reach towards your toes.
- Maintain a steady breathing pattern throughout the exercise.

SUPPORTED SPINE TWIST (60 SEC)

Supported Spine Twist is a great exercise that can help improve your thoracic rotations and alleviate mid back tightness.

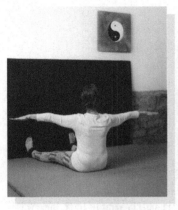
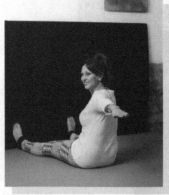
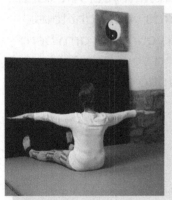
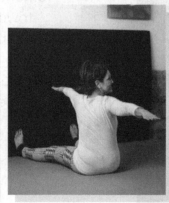

INSTRUCTIONS:

1. Sit tall facing the wall.
2. Straddle your legs and put your feet onto the wall.
3. Extend your arms next to your sides.
4. From this position, rotate your torso towards one side.
5. Rotate your head as well.
6. Repeat on the other side.

COMMON MISTAKES TO AVOID

- Bending the knees.
- Bending the back.
- Rushing the movement.

GENERAL TIPS:

- Inhale at the beginning of the movement and slowly exhale as you rotate your torso.
- Focus on keeping your back straight and your movements slow and controlled.

WALL CRUNCH (60 SEC)

Perform this effective exercise to engage your abs and stretch your back muscles.

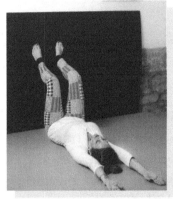
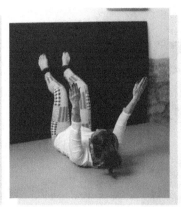
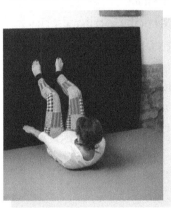

INSTRUCTIONS:

1. Lie flat on your back and place your knees at a 90 degree angle against a wall.
2. Extend your arms backwards beside your head.
3. Tighten your abs and crunch up, bringing your arms forward to touch the floor with your fingers.

COMMON MISTAKES TO AVOID

- Arching your lower back
- Failing to lift your shoulders off the floor.
- Using momentum

GENERAL TIPS:

- Breathe in at the start of the movement and exhale slowly while crunching.
- This breathing technique will increase the activation of your abs.

SIDE TO SIDE CRUNCH (60 SEC)

Side to Side Crunch is a fantastic exercise that will fire up your abdominal muscles, particularly your external oblique muscles.

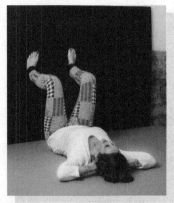
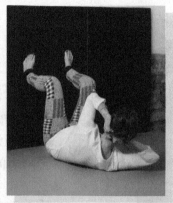
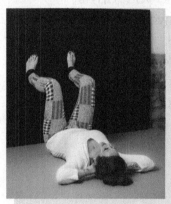
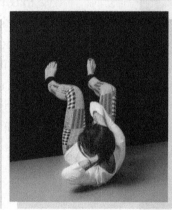

INSTRUCTIONS:

1. Lay flat onto your back.
2. Keep your knees bent on the wall at 90 degrees.
3. Bring your hands behind your head.
4. Tighten abdominals and raise your shoulders off the floor.
5. Crunch your body to one side.
6. Do both sides.

COMMON MISTAKES TO AVOID

- Doing one side only
- Not engaging abdominals
- Rushing the movement.

GENERAL TIPS:

- Inhale at the beginning of the movement, and slowly exhale as you start crunching to the side. This will increase the activation of your abdominal muscles.

REACH THROUGH CRUNCH (60 SEC)

Reach Through Crunch is an effective exercise for activating your abdominal muscles.

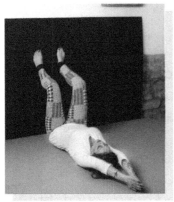 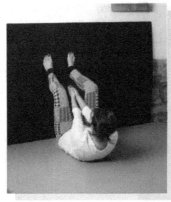

INSTRUCTIONS:

1. Lie on your back with your knees bent at a 90 degree angle against a wall.
2. Extend your arms over your head and place your hands together.
3. Engage your core and bring your hands between your knees.

COMMON MISTAKES TO AVOID

- Arching your lower back
- Not lifting your shoulders off the floor.
- Using momentum.

GENERAL TIPS:

- Inhale at the beginning of the movement and exhale slowly as you crunch.
- Focus on performing the exercise with control and without rushing through the motion.

KNEE TO CHEST (RIGHT) (60 SEC)

Knee to Chest is an effective exercise for activating your hip flexor muscles and building strength in this area.

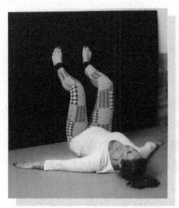 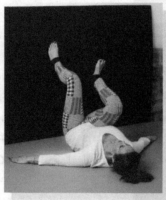

INSTRUCTIONS:

1. Lay flat on your back.
2. Put your knees at a 90 degree angle against a wall.
3. Extend your arms to your sides.
4. Lift and bring your right knee towards your chest..

COMMON MISTAKES TO AVOID

- Moving too quickly
- Holding your breath
- Arching your lower back

GENERAL TIPS:

- Focus on maintaining a steady breathing pattern throughout the exercise.
- Keep your body relax ed and your movements controlled.

LIFTED KNEE TO CHEST (RIGHT) (60 SEC)

This exercise will fire up your glute and hamstring muscles. It is one of the most difficult variations when it comes to bridge exercises.

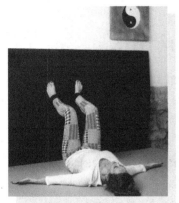 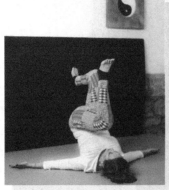

INSTRUCTIONS:

1. Lay flat on your back.
2. Put your knees at 90 degree angle on the wall.
3. Extend your arms to your sides.
4. Push off the wall with your left foot and bring your hips up.
5. While doing that, bring your right knee towards your chest.

COMMON MISTAKES TO AVOID

- Going too fast
- Arching the lower back
- Holding the breath

GENERAL TIPS:

- To prevent any arching in the lower back, gently contract your abdominal muscles.

KNEE TO CHEST (LEFT) (60 SEC)

Knee to Chest is an exercise that can activate your hip flexor muscles and help build strength in that area.

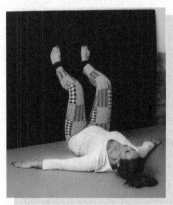 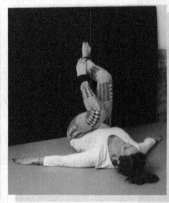

INSTRUCTIONS:

1. Lie flat on your back.
2. Place your knees at a 90 degree angle against a wall.
3. Extend your arms out to the sides.
4. Lift and bring one knee toward your chest.
5. Lower your leg back to the starting position and repeat with the other leg.

COMMON MISTAKES TO AVOID

- Moving too quickly
- Holding your breath
- Arching your lower back

GENERAL TIPS:

- Try to maintain a steady breathing pattern throughout the exercise.
- If it's difficult, focus on exhaling as you bring your knee toward your chest.

LIFTED KNEE TO CHEST (LEFT) (60 SEC)

This exercise will fire up your glute and hamstring muscles. It is one of the most difficult variations when it comes to bridge exercises.

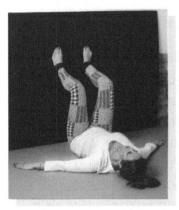 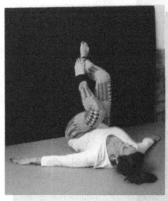

INSTRUCTIONS:

1. Lay flat on your back.
2. Put your knees at 90 degree angle on the wall
3. Extend your arms to your sides.
4. Push off the wall with your right foot and bring your hips up.
5. While doing that, bring your left towards your chest.

COMMON MISTAKES TO AVOID

- Going too fast
- Arching the lower back
- Holding the breath

GENERAL TIPS:

- To prevent any arching in the lower back, gently contract your abdominal muscles.

TABLE OBLIQUE TWIST (60 SEC)

This exercise is a great choice if your plan is to fire up your abdominal muscles. It will work both the side and front parts of the abdominal muscles.

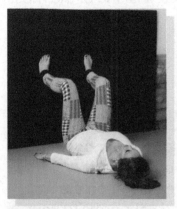 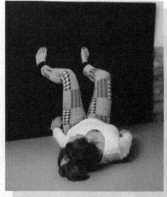

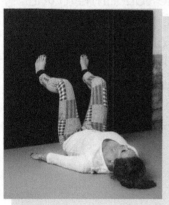 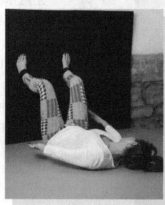

INSTRUCTIONS:

1. Lay flat on your back.
2. Put your knees at a 90 degree angle on the wall.
3. Activate your abdominals and extend your hands forward.
4. Crunch to one side.
5. Crunch to the other side.

COMMON MISTAKES TO AVOID

- Not letting your shoulders off the floor.
- Crunching to one side only.
- Using momentum.

GENERAL TIPS:

- Inhale at the beginning of the movement and slowly exhale as you start crunching. Doing the movement this way will increase the abdominal activation.

OTHER TIPS TO KEEP YOU HEALTHY!

NUTRITION

Nutrition is one of the best ways of preserving your health and overall wellbeing. In America, the incidence of malnutrition ranges from 12% to 50% among the hospitalized elderly population and from 23% to 60% among institutionalized older adults. In the UK, approximately 10-20% of elderly people are at medium-high risk of malnutrition. The effects of malnutrition include:

EFFECTS	CONSEQUENCES
POOR IMMUNE SYSTEM	Impaired ability to fight infection
REDUCED MUSCLE STRENGTH AND FATIGUE	Reduced capacity to work, shop, cook, and take care of oneself due to inactivity. The poor muscular function can lead to falls, and poor respiratory muscle function can lead to low cough pressure, which can delay expectoration and recovery from a chest infection.
IMPAIRED WOUND HEALING	Infections and un-united fractures are more common as a result of increased wound-related complications.
IMPAIRED PSYCHO-SOCIAL FUNCTION	Malnutrition causes apathy, sadness, introversion, self-neglect, hypochondriasis, loss of libido, and worsening in social relations.

Nutrition preserves your health by providing all the nutrients your body needs in order to function properly. The body needs a variety of different nutrients to maintain the health and strength of your bones, muscles, organs, connective tissues and so much more. This is why a balanced diet is so important.

Every nutrient performs a different role within the body, and each nutrient is codependent. This means that if you don't obtain enough of one nutrient, the body will struggle to absorb another. This can create a ripple effect leading to numerous nutritional deficiencies. Then, these deficiencies can cause symptoms like weak bones, tiredness, mood swings, hormonal imbalances, and more.

So, how do you ensure that you eat healthily? The Eatwell Guide sets out food categories and recommendations for all. By consuming a mixture of all food groups, you will consume a variety of nutrients required to keep you healthy.

FRUIT AND VEGETABLES

39% of our total food intake should come from fruit and vegetables. This can be translated into consuming 5 portions of fruit and vegetables per day.

A portion is:
- Approximately 80g of fruit
- 1 whole medium-sized piece of fruit eg. Apple/banana
- 2 small-sized pieces of fruit eg. Satsuma/plum
- 1 large slice of pineapple/melon
- 3 tablespoons of vegetables
- 1desert sized bowl of salad
- 30g dried fruit
- 150mls unsweetened fruit juice
- 150mls smoothie

Fresh, frozen, tinned, and dried fruit all count towards our 5 a day. If you are underweight or you've experienced significant weight loss in a short period of time then tinned fruit in syrup would be more sensible. We should aim to eat a variety of different coloured fruits and vegetables as they contain different antioxidants. The main nutrients provided in fruit include dietary fibre, vitamin C, potassium, folate and vitamin A.

STARCHY CARBOHYDRATES

37% of your total food intake should come from starchy carbohydrates.

Good examples of carbohydrates include:
- Breakfast cereals
- Couscous
- Semolina
- Tapioca
- Bulgar wheat.

Starchy foods should ideally be included at every mealtime. Wholegrain and wholemeal versions should be chosen where possible to help meet your fibre requirements of 30 grams per day. This is especially important for older people due to higher occurrences of constipation. Starchy carbohydrates provide dietary fibre, B vitamins, carbs, and calcium.

PROTEIN

On average, an older person requires approximately 0.75g of protein per kilogram of body weight a day/ However, many adults need 1g of protein per kg of bodyweight. The intake can also be different depending on your nutritional status and weight. Approximately 12-15% of our total food intake should come from this section. Beans, peas, tofu, lentils, and other vegetables are a good source of alternatives to meat as they are low in fat and high in protein, vitamins, and minerals.

It is recommended that adults eat two portions of fish per week, one of which should be oily such as salmon or herring. These oily fish are a valuable source of omega 3 fatty acids which can have a positive effect on memory, heart health and inflammation, and mood.

These foods are a good source of iron, which is essential for making red blood cells that carry oxygen around the body. A lack of iron can lead to iron deficiency anemia. This is common in older individuals as its prevalence increases with age. This can also occur as a result of chronic gastrointestinal blood loss caused by some medications and gut conditions. This type of anemia should be treated with iron supplements. On average an older adult requires 8.7mg per day. Those with a diagnosed deficiency require more and should be managed by a medical professional. This food group provides nutrients like iron, protein, b vitamins, and omega 3 fats.

FATS, SALT, AND SUGAR

Foods high in sugar, salt, and fat such as biscuits, cakes, and soft drinks sit outside the Eatwell Guide. While these foods can be enjoyed in moderation as part of a balanced diet, if eaten regularly they can increase the risk of health conditions such as high blood pressure, obesity, and type 2 diabetes. It is also important to stay hydrated, try to drink 6-8 glasses of fluids daily.

DAIRY AND ALTERNATIVES

8% of your total food intake should come from this section. Milk, cheese, and yogurt are excellent sources of calcium and protein and we should aim to eat 3 portions every day.

Great sources include 200ml of milk, a pot of yoghurt or a matchbox size of cheese as well as calcium-enriched alternative milk like almond, rice and soya. This food group provides nutrients like calcium, protein, vitamin A.

OILS AND SPREADS

Oils and spreads can be high in saturated fats so it's important to minimise these and choose healthier choices. These include plant sources like rapeseed, sunflower, or olive oil. Unsaturated fats are more cardio-protective (heart-healthy) than saturated versions like butter and lard.

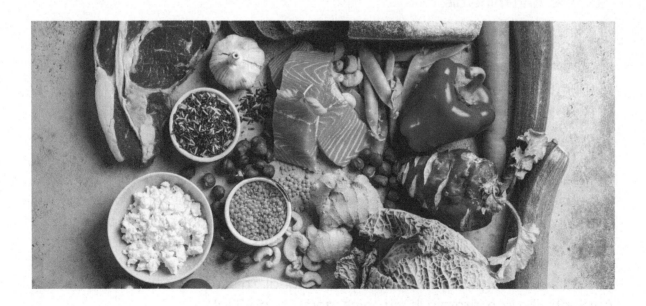

CALORIE AND MACRO REQUIREMENTS FOR OLDER ADULTS

Below is a table that summarises calorie and macronutrients requirements for average persons in different age categories.

AGE	65-74		75+	
NUTRIENT	MALE	FEMALE	MALE	FEMALE
CALORIES	2,342	1,912	2,294	2,840
PROTEIN (G/DAY)	53.3	46.5	53.3	46.5
TOTAL FAT (G/DAY)	91	74	89	72
CARBOHYDRATES (G/DAY)	312	255	306	245
FIBRE (G/DAY)	30	30	30	30

** These are recommended intakes for average persons and can vary based on a persons body composition and health.

VITAMINS AND MINERALS IMPORTANT FOR SENIORS

As we get older, our calorie needs decrease. This means that everything we eat should be packed with nutrients in order to achieve the recommended intake.

There are certain nutrients that are more important than others, especially when we get older.

CALCIUM

Calcium is vital for maintaining healthy bones and teeth. This nutrient can be obtained from dairy products and alternatives.

VITAMIN D

Vitamin D aids in the absorption of calcium, the maintenance of bone density, and the prevention of osteoporosis. Vitamin D has also been shown to protect against cancer, type 1 diabetes, rheumatoid arthritis, multiple sclerosis, and autoimmune illnesses in some studies. Vitamin D insufficiency has also been related to an increased risk of falling in the elderly.

VITAMIN B12

Vitamin B12 is a nutrient that aids in the health of the body's nerve and blood cells, as well as the production of DNA, which is the genetic material found in all cells. Vitamin B12 also protects against megaloblastic anaemia, which causes fatigue and weakness.

OMEGA-3 FATS

These unsaturated fats, which are mostly found in fish, may help with rheumatoid arthritis symptoms and decrease the advancement of age-related macular degeneration (AMD), a disease that causes visual loss in the elderly.

MAGNESIUM

Magnesium is involved in more than 300 different physiological activities. Getting enough can help you maintain a healthy immune system, a healthy heart, and strong bones. Older adults who use certain medications, such as diuretics, may have trouble absorbing magnesium, so a supplement may be beneficial.

FIBER

Fibre is an important nutrient that supports a healthy gut and lowers blood pressure and blood sugar. As you age, you might find that constipation can be a regular problem, obtaining enough fibre may help with this issue.

POTASSIUM

Potassium is an important mineral that helps to maintain strong bones and teeth. This mineral is necessary for cell function and has been found to help lower blood pressure and minimise the chance of kidney stones.

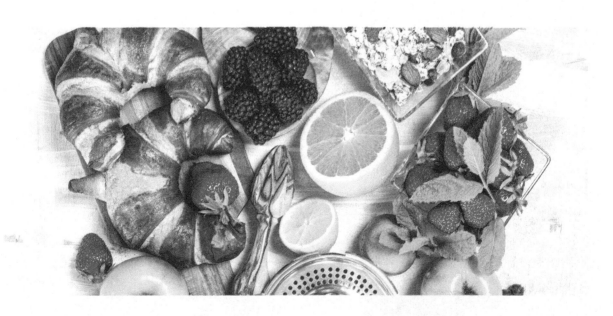

VITAMIN AND MINERAL REQUIREMENTS FOR SENIORS

Below is a table that summarises vitamin and mineral requirements for average persons in different age categories.

AGE	65-74		75+	
NUTRIENT	MALE	FEMALE	MALE	FEMALE
VITAMIN A (MG/DAY)	700	600	700	600
THIAMIN (MG/DAY)	0.9	0.8	0.9	0.7
RIBOFLAVIN (MG/DAY)	1.3	1.1	1.3	1.1
NIACIN EQUIVALENT (MG/DAY)	15.5	12.6	15.1	12.1
VITAMIN B6 (MG/DAY)	1.4	1.2	1.4	1.2
VITAMIN B12 (MG/DAY)	1.5	1.5	1.5	1.5
FOLATE (MG/DAY)	200	200	200	200
VITAMIN C (MG/DAY)	40	40	40	40
VITAMIN D (MG/DAY)	10	10	10	10

** These are recommended intakes for average persons and can vary based on a persons body composition and health.

MENTAL HEALTH

Maintaining good mental health in our golden years is essential for wellbeing and quality of life. Thankfully, there are a number of simple tips and strategies that can be used to help maintain their mental health. In this section of the chapter, we'll look at 10 easy tips for better mental health. From activities to help reduce stress, to tips for staying connected to loved ones, these tips can make a big difference in the lives of seniors.

WHAT IS MENTAL HEALTH ALL ABOUT?

Mental health is about more than simply being free from mental illness. It is about feeling good about yourself, having positive relationships with those around you, and coping with life's challenges in a healthy way. Mental health is an essential part of overall wellbeing, as it enables us to maintain resilience and cope with life's ups and downs. Mental health involves many aspects, including our emotions, thoughts, behaviors, and social connections.

Mental health issues are common in seniors, with approximately one-third of adults aged 65 and older experiencing some form of mental health issue. This can include depression, anxiety, bipolar disorder, Alzheimer's disease, dementia, and more. Additionally, mental health issues can lead to other physical health problems if they are not properly managed.

For seniors, it is especially important to stay on top of their mental health and wellbeing. Regular physical activity, social interaction, and engaging in meaningful activities can all help seniors stay mentally healthy.

BENEFITS OF TAKING CARE OF MENTAL HEALTH

Mental health is an important part of overall wellbeing, and it can become more important as we age. Taking the time to maintain good mental health can provide a number of benefits that can improve quality of life for seniors.

Some of the benefits of taking care of mental health include:
- Increased self-esteem and sense of purpose: Keeping your mind active can give you a greater sense of self-worth and help keep boredom at bay.
- Improved social connections: Connecting with others can help reduce feelings of loneliness and isolation, and make life more enjoyable.

- Reduced stress: Lowering stress levels can reduce anxiety and depression symptoms, as well as improve physical health.
- Enhanced memory and cognitive functioning: Keeping your mind active can help protect against age-related cognitive decline and dementia.
- Improved mood and energy levels: Maintaining good mental health can provide a better outlook on life, as well as increase motivation to complete tasks.

Taking the time to prioritize your mental health can go a long way in providing positive benefits to your overall wellbeing. These benefits may include improved quality of life and better overall physical health.

TIPS FOR BETTER MENTAL HEALTH

GO FOR REGULAR WALKS AND FRESH AIR

Regular exercise is important for physical and mental health, but it can be difficult for seniors to get enough exercise. Going for walks can be a great way for seniors to get the exercise they need and get some fresh air at the same time. Fresh air can do wonders for your mental health and going on a walk can help you clear your head, reduce stress, and improve your mood. If possible, try to walk in a park or other outdoor area with plenty of greenery and nature. This can help you relax and enjoy the scenery while you're walking. For those who have difficulty getting out and walking, joining a walking group may be an option. Walking groups provide companionship, accountability, and encouragement to help seniors get the exercise they need.

GET ENOUGH SLEEP

Sleep is an important part of keeping good mental health, and seniors are no exception. A lack of quality sleep can lead to depression, anxiety, cognitive decline, and many other issues.

The National Institute on Aging recommends that seniors aim for seven to nine hours of sleep every night. However, if you find yourself struggling to stay asleep or get enough restorative sleep, you may need to adjust your sleeping habits.

For starters, try to go to bed and wake up at the same time every day. Create a relaxing nighttime routine by dimming the lights and avoiding screens for at least an hour before bed. It's also important to keep your bedroom cool and comfortable—around 65°F is ideal—and to limit caffeine and alcohol consumption in the evening.

If you're still having trouble sleeping, talk to your doctor about possible treatments, such as cognitive-behavioral therapy (CBT) or medications that may help you get better rest. With the right steps, you can make sure you're getting enough sleep each night and taking care of your mental health.

TAKE BREAKS DURING THE DAY

Taking breaks during the day can help seniors stay focused and keep their mental health in check. Even if it's just taking a few minutes to sit and relax, stepping away from your work or day-to-day activities can be beneficial. Taking a short walk outside, listening to some calming music, or reading a book are all good ways to take a break during the day.

If possible, try to create a set schedule where you can plan regular breaks throughout the day. During these breaks, make sure to step away from screens and electronics and engage in some sort of activity that will help to reduce stress. This could be something as simple as stretching, meditating, deep breathing exercises, or yoga.

If you have a hard time remembering to take breaks throughout the day, try setting a reminder on your phone or computer. You may also want to ask family members or friends to remind you when it's time for a break. Taking time for yourself can help you remain focused and energized for whatever tasks come next.

CONNECT WITH OTHERS

Staying socially connected is important for all of us, especially seniors. Social interaction helps to stimulate the mind and maintain a healthy emotional state. Make time to reach out and connect with friends, family members, and even strangers. This could be as simple as taking a walk around the block and saying hello to your neighbors or joining an online forum. If you are feeling more adventurous, you could join a local club or organization, volunteer at a charity event, or simply make plans to have lunch with an old friend.

No matter how you choose to stay connected, remember that social interaction can be very beneficial for mental health. It helps to increase feelings of belonging, provide support during difficult times, and can even help reduce stress and anxiety. It is essential that we make time in our lives for meaningful relationships and activities that bring us joy and purpose.

DO SOMETHING YOU ENJOY EVERY DAY

It's important for seniors to make time for activities that bring them joy. Doing something you enjoy every day can be a great way to boost your mental health and overall wellbeing. Whether it's reading a book, doing a craft, going for a bike ride, or having coffee with a friend, it's important to make time for things that bring you happiness.

Having an activity that you look forward to every day can be an incredible source of joy and comfort, especially during times when it can be difficult to stay positive. It's also a great way to stay active and social, which are key to maintaining good mental health in seniors.

The important thing is to find something that brings you joy. It doesn't have to be anything big or complicated – it could be as simple as spending 10 minutes playing with a pet, or watching your favorite show. The goal is to do something that makes you feel happy and relaxed, so you can focus on the positive aspects of life.

VOLUNTEER

Volunteering is a great way for seniors to give back and help their community. It can also be beneficial to their mental health by providing a sense of purpose, making them feel needed, and increasing their social interaction. There are many ways for seniors to volunteer. They can choose from local charities and organizations, or even become part of a virtual volunteer team.

For those who are physically able, they can participate in tasks such as gardening, visiting the elderly, or helping with home repairs. For those who are not as mobile, there are still plenty of volunteer opportunities, such as tutoring, fundraising, and working in the office. Whatever their passion may be, there is likely a volunteer opportunity that will fit it.

Another great way for seniors to volunteer is through virtual volunteering. This form of volunteering allows them to stay connected with others while doing something worthwhile from the comfort of their own home. They can participate in activities such as transcribing audio files, proofreading documents, or participating in online surveys.

Volunteering has been proven to have positive impacts on mental health and overall wellbeing. It's a great way to give back while staying active and engaged with the community. With so many options available, there is something for everyone to do.

LEARN SOMETHING NEW

Learning something new is a great way for seniors to stay mentally active and engaged. Taking classes, going to lectures, joining a book club, or reading more can be great ways to explore the world and keep your mind sharp. There are many online courses and educational programs available, as well as in-person learning opportunities. Learning something new can also help seniors stay up to date with the latest technology and trends. Take the time to find something that interests you and commit to learning more about it!

BE MINDFUL OF YOUR THOUGHTS

It's important for seniors to be mindful of their thoughts. The mind can play tricks on us, often leading us to overthink and worry excessively about situations that are outside of our control. When we allow ourselves to be consumed by negative thinking, it can quickly spiral out of control.

Instead, take the time to recognize your thoughts and choose how to respond to them. Remind yourself that thoughts are not facts, and that you have the power to choose which ones to hold on to. Take a few moments to pause and be present in the moment without judgment or expectation. Acknowledge any negative thoughts, but also make an effort to reframe them in a more positive light.

When facing mental health struggles, it can be helpful to seek out professional help from a therapist or doctor. Remember that these issues should not be taken lightly, and there is no shame in asking for support. Mental health issues can affect anyone at any age, so don't hesitate to reach out for help if needed.

Another great way for seniors to volunteer is through virtual volunteering. This form of volunteering allows them to stay connected with others while doing something wortles, it can be helpful to seek out professional help from a therapist or doctor. Remember that these issues should not be taken lightly, and there is no shame in asking for support. Mental health issues can affect anyone at any age, so don't hesitate to reach out for help if needed.

SEEK PROFESSIONAL HELP IF NEEDED

Mental health issues can be difficult to manage on your own, so it's important to seek professional help if needed. Consulting a mental health specialist such as a psychologist or psychiatrist can be beneficial for seniors who are having difficulty coping with emotional challenges. There are also many services available to seniors that provide support, counseling, and other forms of assistance. It is important to remember that seeking professional help is not a sign of weakness, but rather a sign of strength and courage. Taking the steps necessary to get the help you need is an important step in maintaining good mental health.

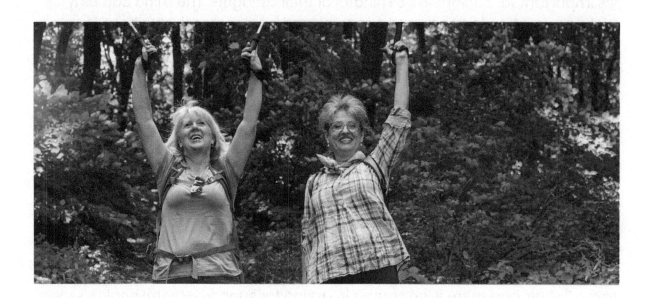

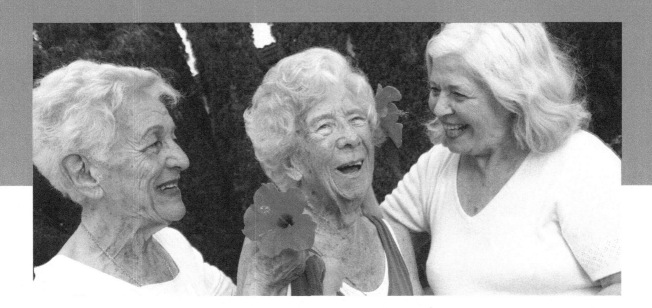

THANK YOU!

At the end of the day, wall pilates for seniors has proven itself to be an invaluable form of exercise that can truly improve the overall health of seniors. Wall pilates can truly be considered a "gift of health" for seniors, enabling them to reach their physical, mental, and emotional goals while having fun and feeling healthier.

Thank you so much for choosing our guide to help you achieve optimum health. We hope you've enjoyed the content!

If so, I have a small request for you.

If you've found value in your reading experience today, I humbly ask that you take a brief moment right now to leave an honest review of this book. It won't cost you anything but 30 seconds of your time—just a few seconds to share your thoughts with others.

If you're reading on Kindle or an e-reader, simply scroll to the last page of the book and swipe up—the review should prompt from there.

If you're on a Paperback or any other physical format of this book, you can find the book page on Amazon (or wherever you bought this) and leave your review right there.

Rita Davis

Made in the USA
Las Vegas, NV
14 August 2024